Quality *14.95*

fatigue factor

Written by

DR. RICK W. GEBHART, D.O.

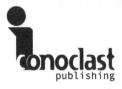

onoclast
publishing

An Iconoclast Book

Published by The Iconoclast Publishing Company

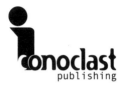

An Iconoclast Book

Published by The Iconoclast Publishing Company

Fatigue Factor
Copyright © 2007 Dr. Rick Gebhart, D.O.
Published by Iconoclast Publishing
Dayton, OH

Contact Information:
Iconoclast Publishing
iconoclast@woh.rr.com

Printed in United States of America
Fatigue Factor
Dr. Rick Gebhart, D.O.
1. Fatigue Factor 2. Dr. Rick Gebhart 3. Medical/Self Help
Library of Congress Control Number: 2006903404
ISBN 10: 0-9779754-0-1
ISBN 13: 978-0-9779754-0-2

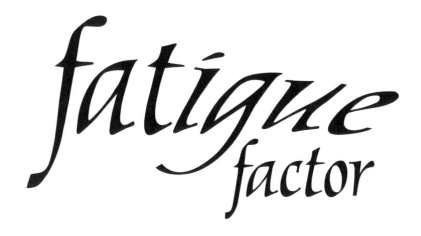

fatigue factor

Written by

DR. RICK W. GEBHART, D.O.

ACKNOWLEDGMENTS

Fatigue Factor is a book written in response to both the debilitating exhaustion I have witnessed in my patients, and the dismal selection of accurate, medical information published to help them. It is my wish that people burdened with fatigue will find easy-to-read yet scientifically plausible answers to their tiredness. Hopefully, I have succeeded in my mission.

This endeavor would not have been possible, of course, without the assistance and generosity of others. I would like to take this opportunity to thank some of these people.

First, I would like to thank all of my fatigued patients who have allowed me to "practice" on them all these years. After twelve years of schooling and finishing my residency, I thought I knew something about medicine. I didn't know squat. Eleven years and seventy-five thousand patients later, I understand a little more. We've learned a lot together over the last decade.

Second, I want to thank my parents. I appreciate and love my father for teaching me that no knowledge is wasted, and my mother for her hands-on learning techniques that kept me a step ahead. I am eternally grateful to them for their inspiration and work ethic, which motivated me to finish this book.

Third, I am appreciative to Dr. Troy Tyner, who read and critiqued this book. If a smarter, kinder physician exists in this world, I would like to meet him.

Thanks to Lisa, my original editor, who led my paragraphs to slaughter, always to cook up something better. Thank you for your dedication and tireless effort.

Lastly, and most importantly, I want to thank my talented and beautiful wife, Tracy, whose cover design graces this book. Thanks for thinking I'm the next Sidney Sheldon and telling me I remind you of Brad Pitt—when I'm not, and…I don't. Luv my baby.

Contents

FORGET WHAT YOU KNOW ABOUT FATIGUE

Modern man's energy drain has been blamed on many things, from the biological burden of budding yeast to the incompatibility of food and blood type. Each new piece of sophistry on the subject amounts to little more than a poorly executed study, supported by a rickety foundation of pseudoscience, designed to prove whatever theory will get you to pay $15.99 for it. Books about fatigue are often full of alluring myths and promises that they alone hold the secret to finding your body's hidden energy. I hate to be the one to break it to you, but believe it or not—sometimes, it just isn't true.

As a board-certified family physician, lecturer, and medical school professor, I am bothered by the charlatanism that sometimes masquerades as science. For twelve years I have diagnosed, treated, and counseled patients with fatigue, and I have seen an overwhelming majority of them get better. However, along the way, I have often had to sit idly by as they shunned my advice, choosing instead to wander through a jungle of worthless over-the-counter potions and magical diets. Yes, a few conditions exist in which herbs, supplements, and vitamins are helpful, but I have found that fatigue typically isn't one of them. After treating more than seventy-five thousand patients in my career, I can only think of a handful of cases where these substances were helpful in alleviating chronic tiredness. Although I occasionally run across a case or two of true vitamin deficiency, what I usually find in low quantities is common sense. Thus, I decided to write this book.

I tell my patients that life is too short to feel bad, and I'm sure that many of you have felt bad for a long time. I just wish that I could sit down with each and every one of you, rest my hand on your shoulder, and hear your story—but I can't. I can tell you that although every condition is not curable, most are at least treatable, and I strongly believe that I can help a lot of you get better. I can guide you logically and scientifically through the medical black forest. Upon emerging from the trees, you should have a clear view of your diagnosis and be able to work towards a solution.

For a long time I have weathered the frustration of seeing so many patients suffer needlessly. I am not a savior, just a mere guide. I strongly believe that I can help a lot of you get better. So, if you are tired of being tired and weary of being weary, kick your feet up on the ottoman and turn the page. We're about to enter the forest.

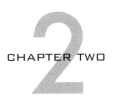

BURST THE MYTH BALLOON

"Doctor, I know my body," many patients say, and though I get a little tired myself when I hear it, I do empathize with them. They are partially right: they know enough about their bodies to realize that something has changed, something has gone wrong. And they come to me—as well as several thousand other doctors, primary care providers, herbalists, dieticians, chiropractors, and pharmacists—looking for answers. Unfortunately, many go away unsatisfied.

In an effort to help their patients, medical consultants frequently run enough blood work to cause anemia, yet in the end, report that nothing is wrong. Herbalists add one more packet of goo-goo weed to the mix, although other than spicing up a roasted chicken, it probably doesn't do much of anything. Chiropractors sell a 39-visit package, and pharmacists point to the "designer vitamin" aisle. But none of them create much energy.

Let's face it, everybody at sometime in his or her life experiences fatigue. We can all find one thing or another to blame for it, like working too much, or running around after the kids. Heck, it's tiring enough just living a normal life. But one mistake that patients make in their critical analysis of what's gone wrong when fatigue sets in is that they view their body as a fixed entity instead of the complex, evolving being that it really is. One day they wake up and realize that they feel bad, and like a car that suddenly doesn't start, they assume a simple part has gone on the fritz. Unfortunately, it's not that easy.

Before I went to medical school, I was an engineering student. Two classes that I had to hurdle in that field were Statics and Dynamics. The first course had to do with forces at rest, such as the weight of a building on a particular steel beam. The second was a study of objects in motion, such as the oscillating forces inside a lawyer's brain as he chases after an ambulance ... or, perhaps a better example would be the forces in an airplane wing as it accelerates down a runway. The point is that the concept of statics is fairly simple, and the math associated with it, relatively easy. However, put an object in motion, make it dynamic, and the forces become complex, with proportionally more difficult math. It is the difference between algebra and calculus, or for those of you not versed in mathematics, chicken nuggets and coq au vin.

What this all translates to is the technical difference between an automobile and the human body. Although in reality, a car is in a slow transformation from a working metal machine to a big pile of rust, it is for the most part static, or unchanging. The piston that drives the engine forward now is the same one that propelled it five years ago. In contrast, your body has changed dramatically in a fraction of that time. In a simple revolution of the earth around the sun, your skin has been replaced dozens of times, your red blood cells have died and been replenished, and your bones have been torn down and rebuilt more times than seedy housing in a bad neighborhood. We are a lot more intricate than we understand. Even if we think that we know our bodies, we probably don't. But as I said earlier, that's not to say we don't know that something is wrong.

This complexity of our physical selves leads to a second problem: how patients conduct their search for a solution to their fatigue. Sometimes when the path to wellness appears intimidating, people look for easy answers—blaming their weariness on thyroid problems, low blood sugar, El Niño, or a host of other intriguing maladies. The starchy articles presented by a frenzy of non-medical journals thickens the delusional stew by duping readers into believing that these disorders are rampant and frequently misdiagnosed. Nothing could be further from the truth. Let's pry open the lid on this barrel of bad information and see what misleading myths are swimming around inside.

Myth #1:
Don't Blame the Thyroid

This small gland in the neck is frequently blamed for a mountain of problems, though in actuality it is more like a pitcher's mound. Endocrinologists, who could also be called thyroid specialists, bang their heads on their desks when asked to test and re-test the levels of this gland's hormone. In a later chapter I will spend more time discussing the physiology of it all, but for now I only wish to share what doctors and endocrinologists chat about across the hospital lunch table: not the relative benefits of Italian dressing over Ranch, but the myth that undiagnosed thyroid problems are commonplace.

Severe thyroid deficiencies can cause fatigue, and I have found my share of them over the last decade. Out of about seventy-five hundred complaints of fatigue I heard in that time, I can count less than forty where a thyroid condition was the culprit. Conversely, I had plenty of other patients in that time-treated for thyroid deficiency—who did not complain of fatigue. Many, however, cheer when I find a low thyroid level (which is called hypothyroidism among us professionals) and blame their weight gain and fatigue on whatever minor lab discrepancy gave them that result. Reality smacks them in the face when I place them on thyroid medicine, and they still remain tired and fat.

Then I'm always questioned about whether or not I gave them the proper dosage, or if the blood work was accurate, or I'm made to look at an article in this great medical journal called "Cosmo," which claims to be able to teach me the nuances of thyroid management and how to make my hair shiny and bouncy. When this happens, I take a deep breath, turn on my prerecorded thyroid speech, and watch the disbelieving scowls walk out of my office. Suffice it to say, a lot of erroneous information exists regarding that gland sitting just south of your Adam's apple. In reality, in most cases, it is just not the cause of your fatigue.

Myth #2:
Don't Let Blood Sugar Bring You Down

Blood sugar is another innocent bystander blamed for a multitude of maladies. Yes, glucose that falls below normal can make you feel bad; there are diabetics, as well as a few non-diabetics, who occasionally lose their sweetness because of it. The important fact to note, however, is that although depleting glucose levels is a common occurrence, it only leaves you feeling weak for a short period of time, usually less than thirty minutes. Even in extreme cases, wherein someone may pass out and experience a longer bout of fatigue, it can always be remedied with a bit of sugar. And it usually won't occur again for several weeks, if at all. Daily fatigue is never, never caused by low blood sugar!

It is reasonable, though, to be occasionally screened for diabetes, especially if it runs in your family. Elevated sugars that run in the greater than 200 range (normal range being 60 to 125) can cause fatigue, along with excessive thirst, excessive urination, and blurry vision. Of course, drinking heavily at the local pub can cause the same symptoms, so make sure you know what you did last night before you run to your doctor screaming about having diabetes. At any rate, blood sugar, thyroids, and the myths noted below will all be discussed at greater length later in this book.

Myth #3:
Just Say No to Epstein-Barr

A third myth is one perpetuated by doctors: we call it the lore of Epstein-Barr. Though this virus does cause 84 percent of mononucleosis cases, it doesn't cause long-term fatigue. As an infectious agent, it can render a person exhausted for three to six weeks, with rarer cases extending out to three months. Eighty percent of the time it is spread through the respiratory tract, and the remainder of the time it is downloaded from another person's lips (you non-medical people may know these two means of infection as breathing and kissing). Epstein-Barr is the scourge of high school and college students alike. Unfortunately in the 1980's, it was erroneously linked to Chronic Fatigue Syndrome, and a million weary passengers jumped on this tired train, convinced that they had found their steam-stealer.

Shortly thereafter, for many reasons, Epstein-Barr was disregarded as a cause of Chronic Fatigue, and the hunt for the real culprit moved on. Many patients, however, didn't. If you are still sailing along with a diagnosis of Epstein-Barr as a source of your fatigue, you should abandon that antique ship, make an appointment with a specialist, and get up to date on what we now know regarding Chronic Fatigue. It is amazing that twenty years after a theory has been proven wrong, some physicians still haven't gotten the memo, and unbelievable that a lot of doctors are still participating in the nonsense and perpetuating the myth.

Myth #4:
Jump Off the Vitamin Bandwagon

The last balloon I wish to deflate is actually an entire collection that's been passed down from one source: the vitamin industry, purveyors of more myths than the Greeks and Romans combined. The difference between the ancient legends and the vitamin industry is that the narratives of the former are harmless and enjoyable. The latter, a multibillion dollar business, gives false hope, selling patients a medicine cabinet full of encapsulated substances that are guaranteed to improve the health of their septic systems and little else. Capitalizing on the notion that most people prefer simple answers, the vitamin industry continues to push out toilets full of mis-leading studies from the well-bulked bowels of their research departments. It is funny, though, how none of their "cutting-edge research" ever seems to land in a peer-reviewed medical journal.

In their defense, I will attest that vitamins can be important. It is well known that certain conditions create a need for vitamin supplementation, such as Crohn's disease, ulcerative colitis, and anorexia nervosa. I would even go so far as to agree that certain vitamins are crucial in the prevention of disease. I certainly prescribe my share of vitamins for a host of disorders—for example, B-12 for pernicious anemia, or B complex for hair loss. In addition, I know that a few vitamins can be used in higher-than-recommended dosages to treat certain illnesses, such as high-dose niacin to reduce elevated fats (triglycerides and cholesterol) in the bloodstream. I also tell patients that they can take a cheap multivitamin if they wish, especially if they feel that their diet is not what it should be.

But these scenarios aside, I cannot recall more than a handful of cases of true vitamin deficiency. And to cause fatigue, the deficiency would have to be bad enough to show up in blood-work and/or a physical exam. Let me repeat, this very rarely happens. Along the same lines, I rarely see mineral deficiencies. Minerals are often prescribed erroneously, and often by those most likely to profit from their sale. A recent edition of The Merck Manual, a well-respected medical text, noted that, "Except for iron and iodine, it is uncommon for elemental deficiencies to develop spontaneously in man, however bizarre the diet." Yet despite this, thousands of charlatans peddle their elemental, mineral-containing wares, and profit greatly from them.

These issues surrounding vitamins, minerals, and their possible deficiencies pose a crucial question: Who is performing and evaluating your lab work? Some chiropractors, herbalists, and naturopaths—people not generally known for their training in blood analysis—are performing blood tests as well as interpreting them. If the thought of these folks doing their own blood studies doesn't scare you, there are minesweeping jobs in Bosnia you may want to apply for!

Why does this phenomenon concern me so much? First, the laboratories used by many of these practitioners are just this side of bogus. A study performed a couple of years ago in a prestigious medical journal sent the same blood to five of these so-called labs. Guess what? They received five different sets of results. One lab said certain minerals were low, while another lab said they were in excess. Often, this blood-work is followed up with a prescription for a few hundred dollars' worth of monthly supplements that go in and out of your intestine faster than it takes the seller to cash your check. The only miraculous relief patients of these practitioners often find is the relief of all things green in their wallets.

Second, even if the blood test is valid (and we have ample evidence in most cases to show that it is not), no one but a trained primary care practitioner or specialist is capable of interpreting the values. Any abnormality found in a lab test could potentially be caused by a multitude of diseases, and only someone trained in the art of medicine is really capable of interpreting the results. I realize that this sounds quite elitist, and I'm not saying that I can give you a blood work diagnosis off the top of my head. Even with my twelve years of schooling and years of practice, I sometimes spend several hours pulling out medical textbooks trying to make sense of lab work. I'm only saying that I wish it were as simple as the chiropractors and herbalists make it out to be. I would certainly get home much earlier at night if it were.

With those myths deflated, I now want to start our journey through the real medical causes of fatigue. I'll follow the advice of a gifted Emergency Room doctor who I was lucky enough to train under during my residency; he said, "Rule out what is going to harm the patient in the next five minutes. Then, rule out what will harm them in the next five hours. After that, rule out what will harm them in the next five days." In other words, I want to make sure that I cover the most mortal issues first, so we will begin with the most devastating illness—cancer—and then work our way through the other causes of fatigue. If you feel that you have already diagnosed what's causing your weariness, you may be tempted to skip past this first section, but I encourage you to invest a small amount of time and use the information therein as a second opinion. I also encourage you to complete this book before racing out and ordering a mile-long list of tests, many of which will be recommended based on your own signs and symptoms. I want to be a good steward of your healthcare dollars, and in an era of runaway health costs, it is reasonable to perform only those tests deemed clinically necessary. On the other hand, life is short and whatever tests are needed to find the source of your fatigue may be prudent to order. Hopefully, this book will help you learn the difference between what tests are necessary for your particular condition, and which ones are not.

RULE OUT CANCEROUS CAUSES

The word "cancer" strikes dread in the hearts of all people. All of us fear it—cancer, that is—and one fourth of us will get it. It's the first word that pops into our heads when our bodies go awry, haunting us each night as the lights go out, the world goes silent, and our heads hit the pillows.

Part of the reason it frightens us so much is because we have very little control over it. We can eat well, work out, refrain from smoking and so on, but still succumb to it. Case in point: the first doctor I hired to join my practice was an energetic young woman who was the epitome of good health, both mentally and physically. She went to church, enjoyed aerobics, and delivered two beautiful children into this world—and subsequently died from breast cancer at the age of thirty-four. The word tragedy didn't even begin to describe the shock and pain her family experienced, or what those of us who worked with her felt when she passed. Nobody should have to endure what she did because of this illness, we all know that. And so we all know that it is perfectly normal to be concerned about the same thing happening to us when unexplained fatigue takes root in our bodies.

So, how do we make sure that a cluster of cancer cells isn't marching across our tissues like a military madman? Thankfully, by the time a cancer causes fatigue, it has usually left behind a few clues, and you should already be aware that there's a problem. Just to cover them briefly, most cancers will generally show signs in your blood work, such as anemia (low hemoglobin), low albumin and protein, and an elevated sedimentation rate, which is a measure of inflammation. Keep that in mind for now; I'll speak more about it in the "putting it all together" section at the end of this book.

If cancer is present in your body, other signs, such as soaking night sweats, unexplained weight loss, and physical exam changes noted by your doctor, should be present by the time fatigue sets in. Always remember to tell your primary caregiver every symptom or change in how you feel, even if it means making more than one appointment to review every symptom. Eighty percent of diagnosis is based on the history of the patient's illness, so don't be afraid of opening your mouth to say more than just, "AAAHHH!" A good exam, a complete list of symptoms, and testing your blood for the above-mentioned levels (along with any other testing your doctor deems appropriate) should be able to detect if it is cancer stealing away your life energy.

A caveat certainly should be interjected here, because there is one common question that everyone wants to ask: Could a person harbor cancer without detection? Unfortunately, the answer is yes. A small group or single cancer cell could have recently developed in any of you reading this text, or in me for that matter, without setting off any alarms. The good news, however, is that a few cells are not causing your fatigue. In fact, cancer cells appear in our bodies on and off throughout our lives, but thankfully our immune systems destroy them before they multiply. And the better news is that for those with fatigue, less than one hundredth of 1 percent of them have cancer as a cause of their tiredness. But just because cancer is so monstrous, and so deserving of special diligence, let's spend a few more pages looking at what it is and where it comes from.

Cancer occurs when dividing cells suddenly lose control and grow at an exponential rate. What causes their sudden acceleration in growth? Well, carcinogens (cancer-causing agents) in the environment, radiation, viruses, and genetic mutations can all individually, or in combination, encourage a cell to lose control of its own growth. The faster the cell reproduces, the faster the cancer grows. How deadly the cancer is depends on in which organ it originated, and how quickly the cancer cells divide, all of which can be determined by examining the cells under a microscope.

Cancer kills by literally sucking the lifeblood from the body. Cells that grow at 500 times the normal rate need 500 times the nutrients. This drain on the system weakens us, and as our energy shunts to the new cells on the block, we waste away—our normal cells are no match for these "super-dividers."

What makes cancer curable is its relative susceptibility to chemotherapy or radiation. Diseases such as testicular and thyroid cancers fall quickly to proper treatment, while cancers spawned from places like the pancreas resist our attacks like Army Rangers. To complicate matters, a few treatment-resistant cancer cells might survive the initial wave of treatment and adapt in the hostile environment of the therapy. Once the siege is lifted—that is, when the treatment stops—this tiny block of resistance explodes in growth and brings the cancer survivor to his knees. Unless this new "super-cancer" can be licked with more potent agents, the patient will succumb.

As medicine progresses, hopefully we can make new strides in learning how to kill cancer cells without killing our healthy cells. Ideas currently in progress include methods of disrupting blood supply to tumors, using everyday viruses to kill the cancer cells, stimulating our own immune systems to attack the cancer, and improving our aim with lethal radiation. But the best way to insure our survival against this dreaded villain is still prevention. First, go to your primary care provider regularly for evaluations based on your age, sex, and family history. A good caregiver can recommend how often the various systems need to be checked (yearly pap smears, etc.).

Second, eat right and exercise. I could write about this topic for a hundred pages, but that is beyond the scope of this book, and would probably make most of you gag anyway. Suffice it to say that keeping your immune system in top-working order—which can be done through diet and exercise—may help you stay free of cancer. You doctor can help you find the type of diet and exercise that is right for you.

In summary, cancer is something that lurks in the back of every mind. But if you haven't lost weight, experienced changes in your blood work, or had an abnormal physical exam, your fatigue is probably not coming from the dreaded "C" word. Remember that many other conditions can cause sweating, weight loss, and abnormal lab work results, so don't panic if you have these signs and symptoms. For now, let's leave cancer behind and elaborate on some of the other conditions that cause fatigue.

CHAPTER FOUR

TAKE A WALK THROUGH THE HUMAN BODY

The flesh and blood of modern man constitutes the most complicated array of intricate, symbiotic systems on this planet. To embark on a guided tour of each system in search of the cause of fatigue may seem, at first, overwhelming. But years of systematic, step by step approaches to my fatigued patients' problems have whittled the process, for me, down to an art form. If your primary care provider doesn't seem to be able to connect the pathological dots, or just doesn't act interested, find yourself a good internal medicine physician and voice your concerns. A good left brain and a list of the right questions should take you a long way!

We will start here with the most critical bodily systems and work our way towards the least deadly. Actually, let's begin with the cardiovascular system—the heart and arteries—because it's important for you to know about the devastating toll vascular disease can take on it if it is not properly diagnosed and treated.

The Cardiovascular System

A patient of eight years came into my office one day, complaining of a two-month bout of fatigue. He was about fifty-five years old and worked for an oil company; each day he climbed a long staircase to the top of an oil tank to take readings. As he sat on my exam table, he admitted that recently, for the first time in twenty years, he'd had to stop halfway up to catch his breath.

I performed a good history and physical, and the only thing that seemed abnormal was the fatigue he experienced while climbing the eighty or so spiraling stairs at his workplace. I sent him for a stress test the next day, which was just an EKG (electrocardiogram, a recording of the electrical voltage in the heart) performed while walking on a treadmill. He flunked it in the first five minutes; forty-eight hours later, he was on the operating table receiving by-pass surgery. With clean arteries feeding his heart, he now whistles his way up the stairs as he did when he was a younger man.

So, what tipped me off to the blockages in his heart, and more importantly, what should tip you off to yours? Is this where your fatigue is coming from? There are clues that can help you confirm or dismiss this frightening condition as the cause of your fatigue.

Heart disease can result from blocked arteries that bring oxygen to the pumping muscle or from a variety of infectious agents. Structural problems, such as bad valves, can also cause fatigue, but by the time this condition exacts its tiring effects, any primary care provider should be able to hear the raging murmur that appropriately corresponds. Those are rarer, so we'll look at those last; let's begin with artery blockage (ischemia) and see if that is what is causing your fatigue.

Cardiovascular disease (the narrowing of one or more heart arteries) can diminish the blood flow to the heart tissue itself and cause fatigue. It can come with or without chest, arm, or jaw pain or the typical symptoms of sweating or nausea—especially in women. For 25 percent of Americans, sudden death is the first symptom of something wrong with the heart. You don't need to be a Nanotech Engineer—what we used to call a rocket scientist—to know that sudden death is a really bad symptom. If you are reading this book and think you have cardiovascular-based fatigue, seek help from your primary care provider IMMEDIATELY!

Now that you know that, keep in mind that heart artery blockages produce at least some type of warning in most patients, though a fair number of people either don't recognize the symptoms or ignore them. Blockages usually, but not always, produce pain in the chest, arm, or jaw which comes on with exertion and diminishes with rest. Women, as previously mentioned, frequently experience more subtle symptoms than men do; the same goes for Diabetic patients. In these cases, determining if coronary artery blockages exist depends on several other factors.

The first and most obvious place to look for risks of heart disease is family history—review your parents, siblings, and other close relatives for a vein of early death or heart problems. If your whole family lived to ninety years of age, it is unlikely that you would die at a third of that age from a heart attack. Second, look at your cholesterol levels to determine risk. If lipids (cholesterol and triglycerides) are in an acceptable range, the chance of having heart disease is reduced. Third, if you aren't a smoker and you manage to get some physical exercise on a regular basis, you already have a lowered risk of heart disease.

But even if you fall into every low-risk category, it is reasonable to perform a stress test now and then, especially if your fatigue comes on as the day progresses and/or worsens with exertion. These are red flags to a good health care professional that an underlying heart problem may exist. Take this recent example: a thirty-nine year old female patient, who I had only seen once before, came to my office complaining of fatigue that became worse as the day wore on. She also remembered, after intense questioning, that she had had an episode of chest burning which was relieved with an antacid. She protested strongly for a while, but finally agreed to a stress test. It came back markedly positive, and she is currently undergoing bypass surgery on two 90 percent blockages of her arteries. Moral of the story? If your fatigue is present when you wake up, it probably isn't coronary artery blockage. If it comes on later in the day and gets worse when you're active, there may be a problem. Either way, if you are in doubt, or have a strong family history of heart problems, get a stress test. Really, what can it hurt?

Our main pumping organ can fail us in other ways that produce fatigue, too. We call this condition heart failure, and it can occur for a variety of reasons, which can be simplified down to two: infectious causes and structural defects. First, let's talk about infection.

Two types of organisms can invade your heart and produce fatigue—viruses or bacteria. Bacteria (organisms that respond to antibiotics) can invade the inner lining of the heart. Named endocarditis, this condition can produce fatigue that lasts for a week, or even months. When I was a first-year resident on emergency room rotation, I was given the case of a thirty-five year old female with fatigue that worsened over six to eight weeks and had increased greatly in the last seventy-two hours. She had been to three emergency rooms that evening; the first two did some basic testing and blew her off. Pressed strongly by this lady's well-to-do husband, our ER doctor decided to admit her for further testing and woke me up at 3 a.m. to perform that grueling task.

My initial thought was that she was the typical suburbanite victim of depression, but her persistence in gaining entrance to a hospital at that late hour made me rethink my position. After three hours—the longest physical exam in my career—I discovered long, red, splinter-like changes under two toenails. With a bit more questioning, I learned that she had recently undergone extensive dental work, and although a cardiologist had told her to always take antibiotics prior to any work on her teeth, her family doctor said otherwise. To make a long story short, this lady had contracted a bacterial infection of her heart lining from the dental procedure. She was placed on six weeks of antibiotics and subsequently improved. Luckily, I haven't seen a case like that since.

So while bacteria can be a kind of hidden cause of your possible heart-caused fatigue, viruses are even less obvious and can fool even the best doctors. They come in two flavors, one that attacks the heart's outside covering (pericarditis) and a more serious condition that invades the heart muscle itself (myocarditis). It is the latter that is harder to diagnose, so let's save that one for last.

Viral pericarditis is a common entity that can strike anyone at any time, especially patients who have had heart surgery in the previous three months. The cardinal symptom is shortness of breath during exertion coinciding with chest pain. It can usually be diagnosed by listening to the heart and hearing a "rub" sound (your doctor will know that one, it's a classic) and can usually picked up on an EKG. An ultrasound can diagnose anything missed by those first two methods. The fatigue that this condition brings usually lasts only for six to eight weeks, but the fatigue of its wicked stepsister, myocarditis, can drag on for years.

If a virus invades the muscle of the heart—that's our friend myocarditis—the condition develops more quietly, sending the patient into a long, slow, debilitating fatigue. Myocarditis doesn't stick out like a sore thumb, as do some of the conditions we've already looked at, and can be overlooked by even an astute physician. It is important to know the typical signs and symptoms of this rare disease to be sure that it's not what's stealing your life-energy, so let's go over those now.

An infection in the muscle of the heart causes a progressive weakness of the body as the pumping chamber loses strength. As the increasingly frail muscle tissue struggles to propel blood through the body, the ventricle (muscle wall) begins to swell under the back-pressure of fluid that isn't getting pumped out. Medicines can help treat this problem, though many times the diagnosis is missed for several months. Although the body will eventually destroy the virus, the heart doesn't usually return to normal without treatment. Early diagnosis is important for a faster recovery.

The diagnosis of this disease can be made sometimes from an EKG, usually from a good listen to the heart (if late in the condition), and almost always from an ultrasound. Abnormal extra beats, which physicians are trained to hear through their stethoscopes, are the hallmark echoes of pump failure. However, as previously mentioned, they may not be heard in the disease's early stages, and even an EKG and ultrasound may be negative. However, by the time a significant, persistent fatigue is present, one of these tests should show the cause. If you don't have faith in your primary care provider and have shortness of breath during exertion or other symptoms besides fatigue, seek out a cardiologist and get the right testing done, right away.

Structural defects are the last reason for heart failure that we will look at here. This includes bad valves, thyroid conditions, amyloidosis and sarcoidosis (abnormal protein deposits in the heart wall), and hypertrophic cardiomyopathy (a thickening of the heart wall due to a hereditary condition). By the time these conditions cause fatigue, they all should be readily diagnosable through the stethoscope, EKG, or ultrasound. Rounding out this showcase of abnormalities are electrical problems within the heart, which add up to abnormal rhythms that make the heart beat ineffectively. Patients usually feel these abnormal beats, along with a shortness of breath, and the changes can be picked up on a 24-hour EKG.

Although heart problems are a somewhat rare cause of fatigue, it is critical to rule out these maladies because of the relative seriousness of each. A CRITICAL POINT: Every heart disease that causes fatigue also causes shortness of breath. A good listen to each valve and an EKG are virtually standard for a fatigue work-up, adding an ultrasound if necessary. As I've said before, if you don't have faith in the expertise of your primary care provider and you have fatigue AND shortness of breath, seek out an internal medicine specialist or cardiologist for a second opinion.

The Respiratory System

Pulmonologists, or lung doctors, have two main items locked into their fields of vision. First is the study of the lungs and their conditions; second is the study of sleep disorders. Lung conditions can certainly cause tiredness, but a shortness of breath almost always coincides with fatigue not matter what the overall cause. This is not true of sleep disorders, which cause a patient to wake up as fatigued as when they went to bed. We'll look at the sleep disorders a little further down—for now, let's look at the lung conditions.

Doctors can easily check your lung function with a fairly cheap and simple approach, and I recommend this because I am ... well, cheap and simple. First, listening to the lungs for the absence of fluid or wheezing and the presence of good air movement is essential and uncomplicated—it's done with a stethoscope, no fancy machines necessary. In addition, most doctors have something called a pulse oximeter in their office, which is a device that measures oxygen levels in the blood with an infrared beam. I always measure the patient's level both at rest and after a short walk down the hallway to see if it drops with exertion. Normal levels are 97 to 100 percent for non-smokers and can dip down to 93 percent in those long-term nicotine puffers; levels below 93 percent while at rest generally can cause fatigue. If you seem short of breath and your caregiver doesn't give you the pulse oximeter test, one can be easily performed at your local hospital or outpatient center.

Two other simple tests that can be performed on the lungs are the chest x-ray, a critical element of any fatigue work-up, and pulmonary function studies. The pulmonary function studies are tests that measure the functional capacity of the lungs, and I don't order these tests routinely unless the patient's fatigue comes with a significant shortness of breath.

X-rays, however, are an important element because they are used to look for certain cancers and asymptomatic diseases, as well as at the functioning of the heart. They can discover or rule out diseases such as tuberculosis, cancer, or sarcoid (which causes the body's immune system to become activated for unclear reasons). X-rays could also find paraneoplastic syndrome (Latin for really bad and really expensive), in which fatiguing chemicals are released from an existing cancer, frequently in the lungs. Its chief aggressor, Eaton-Lambert Syndrome, is a rare condition that derives from small-cell lung cancer, causing a debilitating weakness. Thankfully, these are fairly rare. I've only seen two cases of them in my career.

But let's leave all that lung talk behind. The topic of sleep disorders is more important to our conversation on fatigue. Although neurologists and internists occasionally man the sleep lab, lung doctors are frequently at the helm. Two very common (and very commonly missed) sleep disorders come to mind that you should try to rule out in your search for the cause of your fatigue.

The first is narcolepsy, a disease that causes a person to drop off to sleep, or near-sleep, without control. It was at first thought to be caused by boring ministers and lame English lit teachers, but was later recognized as a true medical malady. Narcoleptic patients jump directly to REM (rapid eye movement) sleep, without the usual preceding sixty minutes or so of non-REM sleep. This condition can usually be detected in a sleep study and with two blood tests (called HLA antigen). It should be noted that 25 percent of patients (tired or not) test positive for these antigens, so the blood-work is not the absolute last word on your diagnosis in this case without the blessings of a sleep doctor.

Nighttime studies will also diagnose a second and more common illness, called sleep apnea, a condition I see frequently in my office. This disturbance of breathing while you sleep can be triggered by two different mechanisms. The first, obstructive sleep apnea, is just what it sounds like: the airway is blocked by a thickness of tissue at the back of the throat. This excessive deposit obstructs the airway while you sleep, just after your respiratory drive weakens in the deepening stages of slumber. By the time you get into the deep sleep state—the only truly worthwhile sleep—the shallow pull of your diaphragm as you breathe can't overcome the weight of the obstruction. This effectively stops your breathing and causes your blood oxygen levels to drop.

When it reaches a danger point, alarm bells sound in your body, you go back to stage one sleep again, and the diaphragm pulls a deep, snorting breath. Then, the cycle starts over again. After the night is up, you know you have been asleep, but the worthless stages you accomplished leave you as tired as when you first put your head on the pillow.

A second type of sleep apnea, central sleep apnea, is not caused by obstruction, but rather by a dysfunction of the deepest part of the brain— the medulla. As you fall further into sleep, the signal that tells the diaphragm to breathe originates from a deeper and deeper place in the brainstem. If, during the critical periods of sleep, the medulla doesn't call out for enough breath, those alarm bells sound, and you wake back up to a lighter, worthless stage of sleep. No matter how long you sleep, you wake up as tired as you were when you went to bed.

Every tired patient who cannot find a reason for her weariness needs to have a sleep consult, especially if she snores. If your caregiver refuses to send you to a sleep lab, remind him that you know where and when he plays golf and that his pager number is accessible on the Internet. If that doesn't work, call a local sleep lab and ask for a consultation with a sleep doctor. And if all else fails, tape record yourself at night and replay it in the morning to find out if you can hear your breathing stop during periods of snoring.

In summary, sleep disorders are common and can cause debilitating fatigue. They can be readily treated, once properly diagnosed. Lung disorders cause a lot fewer cases of fatigue, but should be considered if you tend to become short of breath.

The Blood System

Blood is the quintessential river of life that nourishes the trillions of cells that make up our bodies. As incredibly complex as it is, with a thousand things held in critical balance, I am forever amazed at how stable it remains and how the body corrects for abnormalities. Still, miraculous though it is, the blood can be responsible for fatigue, and in this section, I will try to cover the testing necessary to find out if this is where your problem lies.

Anemia, a lack of hemoglobin in the bloodstream, leaps to everyone's minds when fatigue is mentioned. It can be caused by dozens of things, and it comes in three different varieties. Megaloblastic anemia makes the red blood cells big, fat, and red—which might seem like a good thing, but trust me, it's not. This condition usually accompanies the various diseases that also cause deficiencies in vitamin B-12 or folic acid; if a first blood test shows megaloblastic anemia, levels of B-12 and folic acid should be measured on follow-up blood testing. Sometimes when the tests are normal, patients will ask me for a B-12 shot anyway, and though I don't know if it really helps, patients do seem to get a week or so of boosted energy from it. Also keep in mind that if your blood shows abnormal B-12 or folic acid levels, the intestines should be checked via colonoscopy to find out why these critical substances aren't getting absorbed.

Microcytic anemia creates small, pale red blood cells in contrast to the fat, red ones of megaloblastic anemia. The immature red cells of microcytosis can signify low hemoglobin caused by either a bleeding problem somewhere in the body (usually in the intestinal system), an inability of the marrow to make red cells, or poor iron absorption.

Another type of anemia to discuss is the normochromic type, which has red cells of normal size and color. This anemia features a decrease in hemoglobin, and it is often called an anemia of chronic disease, because it is a slow, gradual process caused by stressful conditions on the body. What isn't a stressful condition to the body, you ask? Well, specifically, we're talking about problems such as brittle diabetes, some cancers, and chronic lung disease, just to name a few. This anemia is rare in people younger than fifty years of age. And thankfully, in most cases, it is mild enough that it doesn't have to be treated, and it doesn't cause fatigue.

Hereditary anemias, from sickle cell (which occurs in African-Americans) to thalassemias (seen in people of Greek descent), round out the field. Any anemia can be diagnosed with a complete blood count—which is the test that looks at red and white blood cells. Though usually read by an electronic counter, abnormal results can be double checked manually by a pathologist with a microscope. Treatment will be based, of course, on what is causing the anemia. Though a slew of people come through my office door convinced that they have anemia for sure, I thankfully find it in only about one in a hundred blood tests. And even then, many cases are mild and not at the root of the patient's fatigue. But because the complete blood count is so easy to perform, it is a necessary test for every fatigued patient.

So we've looked at the red blood cells—now let's concentrate on the white ones. Five types of white blood cells exist: Neutrophils predominate, increasing when needed to fight off bacterial infection. Steroids (medical, not bodybuilding) can raise the level of these cells, as can different types of leukemia. Lymphocytes are the next most common white cell, their excessive number usually caused by viruses, as well as by lymphomas (cancers of the lymph system). Lymphocytes, along with monocytes, the third kind of white blood cell, secrete cytokines, which are mediators of the immune system.

Basophils are the fourth type of white cell found in the blood. Although they also function in the body's immune response to disease, they don't normally increase in number when fighting diseases, so they don't mean much when we're searching for causes of fatigue. Eosinophils, on the other hand can elevate in a variety of conditions. This fifth type of white blood cell can increase in the presence of allergies, parasite infections, cancers, and connective tissue diseases (we'll look at those later, in the rheumatology section of this book). Abnormal levels of this white blood cell are typically blamed on allergies, but if your eosinophil count is raised and you're complaining of long-term fatigue, your doctor should perform a more thorough investigation to find the cause.

Lastly, let's talk about infections before we leave the blood system. Infections can cause fatigue either through the ravages they leave on the body, the toxins that they release, or both. Though short-term infections (for example, pneumonia) cause a white cell count elevation that can be seen in a blood test, long-term infections may not be quite so detectable. Sometimes, the subtlety of a low-grade, chronic infection just doesn't fire up the reaction of the immune system. The only way to detect it is to perform a blood culture, where bacteria are grown in the blood, in a lab, and identified. The specific type of bacteria that grow usually tells the physician where the infection started, which is the first step toward getting rid of the thing that might be causing your fatigue. So keep in mind, if you're a fatigue patient with night sweats or low-grade fevers—both signs of infection, getting a couple of blood cultures done may be of help to you in the long run.

The Gastrointestinal System

In making the transition from blood to guts, our work gets a little simpler. The gastrointestinal system (we'll call it GI from now on, just to save some typing) is certainly less complicated than the confusing world of anemia. It encompasses the biliary system (the gallbladder and liver) as well as the intestinal system, which starts at your mouth and ends up at another orifice that no one likes to talk about in polite conversation. Although you might be tempted to pass this section by, I encourage you not to, because even if you think that you have no gut-related symptoms, conditions could be present that you don't know about. I would hate for you to miss a critical clue on our walk through the body. If it makes you feel any better, I promise to keep the discussion of flatulence to a minimum.

The first thing that comes to mind when I think about GI-related fatigue is the liver. It is an integral part of the digestive process, filtering out toxins and secreting bile to assist in fat absorption. Inflammation of this organ can readily produce fatigue and comes from a variety of sources.

Viral infection of the liver is the most common reason for its inflammation, and the culprits are infections called Hepatitis. The word Hepatitis is generally followed by a letter, A through G, which designates the severity of the infection. Hepatitis A is an acute (rapid and short) infection picked up through things like bad seafood or poor hand-washing; it can make you pretty ill, but it doesn't cause lasting fatigue.

Hepatitis B and C, however, can cause long-term energy depletion. Both can be acquired through blood transfusions that occurred before 1986—screening processes weren't quite so efficient back then; dirty needles; sexual intercourse; and contamination of body fluids. Alcoholics also tend to develop hepatitis C even in the absence of the above. Hallmark signs of both B and C are fatigue and abnormal liver enzymes in the blood, which can be picked up in routine tests.

Hepatitis D through G also exist, but aren't important causes of long-term fatigue in North America or Europe. So instead, I'll instead take this paragraph to mention HIV, which has similar methods of transmission as hepatitis. Any patient with fatigue and the risk factors mentioned above should also get an HIV test. You know, just to be on the safe side of things.

But back to hepatitis. It can also be caused by non-infectious causes, meaning, you don't necessarily have to come in contact with someone else's contaminated fluids to get it. Excessive iron and copper storage, known as hemochromatosis and Wilson's disease respectively, can damage the liver and release enzymes into the blood. In addition, the body can attack the liver just for the hell of it, a condition called autoimmune hepatitis. A liver enzyme panel, which is standard on a chemistry-profile blood test, can screen for all of these diseases. And any of them, regardless of cause or method of infection, can cause long-term fatigue.

Downstream from the liver, diseases of the bowel such as Crohn's disease and ulcerative colitis can produce chronic weariness, but they also produce weight loss and severe diarrhea. If you have one of those conditions, you'll be using the bathroom ten to twenty times a day, and the resulting loss of nutrients from your body will cause fatigue.

Colon cancer, however, may cause fatigue before the diarrhea even begins. Thankfully, it is rare before age forty, though not unheard of, so don't completely rule it out. A good screen for this disease is called fecal occult blood testing, where stool samples are checked for hidden blood. This test should be performed on anyone after age forty, or in younger patients who experience unexplained bowel changes. Any positive testing should be followed with a colonoscopy. And remember, as mentioned previously, cancers usually cause fatigue only after they cause weight loss, so don't panic if your only problem is that you did "number two" a few extra times this week.

A much less serious group of bowel disorders exist, called malabsorption syndromes. As the name implies, these conditions have as their hallmark an inability of the bowel wall to absorb nutrients. Though too numerous to mention all by name, these diseases all show symptoms of diarrhea and weight loss, not to mention abnormally low levels of the various proteins that come standard on chemistry panels in blood work. If these levels are within normal limits, don't worry, because your bowel is probably not the cause of the fatigue.

Moving upward in the body, esophogeal and stomach cancers are thankfully rare in the United States. With these conditions, as with other cancers, weight loss, sweats, and abnormal lab studies usually precede fatigue. And these two GI cancers are usually the result of nicotine and/or alcohol abuse. A test called a barium swallow or upper GI test can usually detect trouble in these areas.

The last place we'll look in this section is underneath your liver, at a little green organ called the gallbladder. This oblong, muscular sack is responsible for spitting out concentrated bile into the small intestine. (And you thought your job was bad!) Fatigue can arise out of the gallbladder in the form of a hidden infection, something which can fool even the brightest of physicians. The following humbling story makes my point.

A pleasant, fifty year old patient came to see me after her regular doctor of thirty-five years retired. She'd complained to that doctor of left shoulder pain that had kept her from sleeping in bed with her husband. Six consultants, three MRI's, two shoulder-scopes and thirty-some odd years later, she was no better. I took this as a challenge, and without boring you with the details, diagnosed the cause of the shoulder pain in less than two weeks. Once better, the patient responded with accolades that would tease any physician into believing that he is ... well, somebody special. But as they say, pride cometh before a fall.

A year or so later, she returned with a complaint of fatigue. I smiled a wry smile, informing her smugly, "You've come to the right place." But two years and seven thousand dollars' worth of tests later, I was scratching my head, her fatigue a complete mystery to me. A top-notch internist contributed another wave of testing and another deep ding in her insurance company. Our expensive work up was only marking time, though, and our lack of success was showing on the tired face of our patient.

At one point, while I was on vacation, she came in to my office complaining of a new pain underneath her ribcage, on the right. When my partner pushed firmly on her gallbladder, it practically sent her jumping off the exam table. By the time I returned, the patient's bile-spitting organ had been removed, along with the long-standing fatigue. She returned back to normal, though she'd lost a couple of years to the gnawing weariness of a hidden infection. Because she'd had no GI complaints, no one had looked at her gallbladder. But once the fatigue showed its ugly face, tests concluded its source.

Pain under the ribcage, frequent nausea, and/or intermittent diarrhea with fatty meals all beg for a gallbladder work up. The first test to do is a simple ultrasound to look for stones, and the second is called an HIDA nuclear scan to test the gallbladder's function. The latter test found the dying organ in my patient.

Because I promised to keep this chapter short, I will end it by mentioning that although not a common source of fatigue, the GI system can be a cause and shouldn't be overlooked. Except for a colonoscopy, your primary care provider should be able to provide most of the testing for the conditions we've covered here.

The Neurological System

One of the most common forms of fatigue that I see comes with a variety of other symptoms, such as dizziness, numbness in the hands, feet, and face, and episodes of passing out. People who have these symptoms call their neurological system into question, wondering if they have a brain tumor or are experiencing symptoms of a stroke. Usually, I get to break the good news to them regarding their benign, or non-life threatening, symptoms.

But how can you know if your body is experiencing a real neurological problem? And how can you find out if your fatigue is coming from the complex array of neurons and gray matter trapped between your eardrums? Having a working knowledge of the brain's anatomy can certainly help calm your fears about what is happening medically in your head. So let's take a look at how this system functions and see how it can inject weariness into your life.

God, I believe, has a dry sense of humor—which explains why He made is so that the right side of the brain controls the left side of the body, and vice versa. But—and this is a very big but—the right side of the brain controls the right side of the face and the temperature fibers for the right side of the body—at least on Tuesdays and Thursdays. Okay, I'm joking about that last part, but the crossover of all fibers except face and temperature, that part is true. Therefore, when a patient tells me that her face, arm, and leg are all numb on one side or the other, I know that this is not a tumor, stroke, or any pathology born of neurological catastrophe. No brain lesion, tumor, or stroke could produce these symptoms. The numbness would have to be in the face on one side, and the arm and leg on the other.

The diseases of the brain and nervous system that are capable of producing fatigue are limited to a handful of conditions, all of which can be corralled into a manageable group. I will do my best to tie them together, based on some universal similarities of the diseases, in hopes that any neurological disease causing your fatigue will stand out.

The first thing to know about neurological disease, as it relates to chronic tiredness, is that the fatigue it produces is a genuine weakness of the arms, legs, and body. Patients often tell me that they are weak, but in reality, their muscle tone is fully intact. So, how do we tell the difference between tired muscles and weak muscles? First, check your reflexes, which always become abnormal before the muscles become weak. Simple knee jerks are the most fragile apparatus of the neurological system, believe it or not, so they will often fall victim to illness before the nerves begin to falter.

Reflexes also tell doctors a lot based on how aggressively they respond to the tap of the hammer. Overly excessive responses indicate problems inside the brain and spinal cord. Poor responses point to trouble outside the central nervous system, in the peripheral nerves. Normal responses don't rule out every neurological disease, but a complete neurological exam usually does. For the most part, primary care providers can perform a good neurological exam in about six or seven minutes and rule out a disease of this system. Thankfully, like some of the other systems we have encountered, they cause less than one hundredth of one percent of persistent fatigue cases.

The Musculoskeletal System

This chapter is dedicated to doctors who proudly don't carry stethoscopes—the orthopedists. Orthopedist comes from two Greek words that mean "players of golf." These champions of bone and muscle carpentry bring the tools of the trade that bear on the human structure—the standards being a hammers and fiber-optic scopes, and thankfully, they see very few cases of fatigue borne out of their domain. And if they did, they would probably just prescribe anti-inflammatories, a handful of Vicodin, and a prescription to play more golf. But I digress...

Besides the various rare bone and muscle cancers (which will be covered in another chapter) and the rheumatological conditions (also discussed elsewhere), only two musculoskeletal ailments cause fatigue. One is a disease of bone and the other of muscle. I will start with the former, called Paget's disease, a condition that afflicts older men and women.

In this destructive disease, cells that normally break down bone so that it can be "remodeled" work overtime, weakening the bones and causing painful, bony lesions. Men dominate this disease condition by a ratio of three patients to two, and once the disease has set in deeply, fatigue can result, as well as heart failure. By the time a patient suffers from the drain on his body that this disease causes, the pain is immense. If the telltale symptoms are not enough, diagnosis can be made by measuring alkaline phosphatase levels in the blood or by performing x-rays or a bone scan. If your bones ache deeply, you are over age sixty, and you are fatigued, get a set of x-rays and an alkaline phosphatase level measured from your blood.

Now, on to diseases of the muscles. Besides the cancers and rheumatological conditions discussed elsewhere, fatiguing illness of the muscles can be reduced to one ailment—muscular dystrophy. MD comes in many forms and attacks various parts of the muscular system. Rather than listing all of them here, I will focus only on the one type of MD that strikes adults.

Most other forms of this condition hit patients by age twenty, usually earlier. Limb-girdle MD, however, can be the problem in adults with weakness (as opposed to tiredness) and atrophy or shrinkage of the hip, chest, and shoulder muscles. Fatigue can also be present in this illness, but not without a noticeable decline in muscle mass. If any doubt exists, a muscle biopsy can be performed to check the diagnosis. Additionally, EMG (needle testing) recordings will generally be positive as well.

Lastly, a quick note should be said about myositis, an inflammation of muscles that can make a patient tired and hurt. This condition can be diagnosed with a blood test, called a sed rate, or if the diagnosis is in question, a muscle biopsy. Thankfully, it is rare.

Before we leave the topic of musculoskeletal illnesses, I want to remind those of you dealing with muscle, joint, or connective tissue pain that a review of the rheumatological system in the next section of this book is a must-read. I see hundreds more of these conditions than I do Paget's or MD, so I encourage you to stay on our walk through the human body a bit longer. I promise to help you find the cause of your tiredness and point you to some answers that will help you get your strength back. But for now, let's jump back into the body.

The Rheumatologic System

Volumes have been written on how the body falls prey to its own immune system, but I will try to keep our discussion of it here fairly brief. I will begin by introducing fibromyalgia, a nonimmune disease that has haunted rheumatologists—doctors who diagnose and treat arthritis and other diseases of the joints, muscles and bones—for years. Fibromyalgia is a condition that has no specific test to diagnose it, only subjective criteria to gauge improvement. It is quite difficult to treat, as the cause is still a medical mystery. Call us crazy, but we doctors prefer illnesses that we can see in lab test results or under a microscope.

Whether health professionals like the disease or not (personally, I enjoy taking care of fibro patients) this condition is a biological thorn—no, make that a spear in the sides of its sufferers. It is one of the most common causes of debilitating fatigue that I've seen, and many of its sufferers have either been misdiagnosed or, more often, gone undiagnosed. For these reasons, it is paramount that we review the clinical features of this condition and see if it might be the cause of your unexplained fatigue.

Fibromyalgia Syndrome, which from now on we'll call FMS, is a disease that is undoubtedly genetic in nature, turned on by a trauma at some point in the afflicted person's life. It is unknown why this condition comes alive after a physical or mental insult, but virtually every patient I encounter with FMS has suffered in one way or another, a year or more prior to the onset of the illness. In many cases, more than a decade has passed between the upsetting event and the start of the disease. This event triggers a disruption in the balance of lower brain neurotransmitters, especially serotonin and norepinephrine, causing the hallmark symptoms of pain and fatigue.

Discomfort in the underlying tissue of the neck, back, arms, and legs, along with debilitating tiredness, are the most consistent complaints that I hear from fibromyalgia patients. Depression, dizziness, and insomnia round out the other common symptoms. Besides the neurotransmitter loss (see Chapter Six for more on that), some researchers believe poor circulation of the cerebrospinal fluid (CFS) could also be to blame. Another factor that contributes to FMS may well be hormonal imbalance. With all of these symptoms, in addition to severe fatigue, draped heavily on these patient's shoulders all the time, is it any wonder they're tired and sore?

So, how do you tell if you are suffering from FMS? Strict criteria are used to make the diagnosis, but I can try to simplify the process for you here. First, you need to be fatigued. I suppose most of you have this symptom, or you wouldn't be reading this book. Second, you should be experiencing tenderness in your neck, upper back, arms, and legs; this pain should be in the tissues and not over or in the joints. Many people with this condition claim that it even hurts when their loved ones touch their skin.

Other symptoms such as insomnia, depression, dizziness, and easy bruising may come with the pain and fatigue. Eighteen potential tender areas on your body can be pointed out by most primary care providers, and diagnosis usually asks for you to have problems with at least eleven of them—although I am more liberal with my counting when there are other symptoms present as well. These points are on your neck, your shoulders, between your shoulder blades, on your upper arms, and on your outer thighs, although many patients have dozens of points all over.

The final "test" for FMS—remember, it has no blood or tissue testing—is to make sure that you don't have another disease causing your symptoms. Bacteria and viruses can make your tissues ache, as well as other rheumatic conditions that show up in the blood. A simple set of lab tests, including a rheumatoid profile, and a CT scan of the head, can rule out any other illness. And before I move on from fibromyalgia, I'll warn you that not all physicians believe in this disease. If yours doesn't and you think you may have it, realize one thing—your doctor is practicing 1960's medicine. Buy him a lava lamp as a parting gift and go find a new physician!

Although fibromyalgia makes up ninety-five percent of the rheumatic conditions causing fatigue, a few others should be noted. The other five percent fall under the heading of autoimmune diseases and might be better described as "friendly fire" conditions in the body. In these instances, our defenses, because of genetic disturbance, lose their ability to distinguish between self and non-self, resulting in an attack on the body's tissues. When the body fires on its own joints, it is called rheumatoid arthritis. When it attacks the joints and the blood vessels, it is termed systemic lupus. Occasionally, the body's defenses will assail the tissues, giving a patient the symptoms of fibromyalgia, but this is actually called mixed connective tissue disease. The two conditions have similar symptoms but are treated completely differently, so make sure that you—and more importantly, your doctor—know the difference.

And how can you possibly tell them apart? With testing, of course. Mixed connective tissue disease is differentiated from FMS by a positive antinuclear antigen blood test and an elevated sedimentation rate (a measure of inflammation—I mentioned that test back in Chapter Three). When the body attacks itself, it leaves certain "footprints" in the bloodstream. ANA, the antinuclear antigen, is a marker of immune response against the body and the hallmark screening test to confirm or deny a rheumatologic disorder. It is normal in FMS, but not in connective tissue disorder. So, there's one way to tell.

Another way is by doing a test called an erythrocyte sedimentation rate, or sed rate, as doctors call it. Also known as ESR, it is a common test ordered to screen for autoimmune conditions and measure the amount of inflammation in the body. FMS, not being an inflammatory condition, will show blood tests with a normal ESR. Rheumatologic conditions such as rheumatoid arthritis and systemic lupus, however, raise the ESR as the body beats up on itself. Infection, cancer, and other conditions can also raise the ESR, so a CBC test (that stands for Complete Blood Count—I know you've heard that one on any given hospital TV show) is usually ordered as well to help determine the cause the cause of the elevation.

Additionally, autoimmune disorders carry their own genetic markers in the blood. Often, though, the mixed cases appear, and a specialist is needed to sort out the conflicting data. If you hurt in your joints, tissues, or both, get tested for these autoimmune conditions. Both FMS and the rheumatologic disorders can cause fatigue, so you never know—they just might be what are behind your ongoing tiredness.

The Immune System

When the body isn't attacking our joints or tissues, it can make us fatigued by wreaking havoc on us immunologically (that's a fancy word for, "via the immune system"). Allergies, a very common complaint, are a dysfunction wherein our body's immune system actually overprotects us. Although this overreaction can make us tired, many things have been blamed on allergies, and not all of that blame is accurate. In reality, allergies share responsibility for only a tiny fraction of the body's problems. To clear things up, let's take a closer look at the types of allergies that assail the human body.

Environmental allergy offenders include grasses, molds, and at least sixty other particulate substances that evoke an immune response from our bodies. Symptoms are usually respiratory (sneezing and wheezing) or dermatologic (itches and rashes). Moderate to severe environmental allergies can give us temporary fatigue as the symptoms flare up, but they can't cause long-term fatigue. Additionally, constant exposure to allergens (for example, working in a moldy building) can make us ill with respiratory infections, but they don't bring on constant, butt-kicking fatigue.

Recently, some experts have tried to link food allergies to fatigue, removing a multitude of things from our diets in an attempt to bring back a our energy. Can food allergies really make us tired? Well, probably not.

The only thing that gastrointestinal allergies gives us are ... you guessed it, gastrointestinal symptoms, and by that I mean stomachaches and good old-fashioned gas. Only secondary infections or dehydration from diarrhea will cause fatigue, and even then, it's only temporary. So, why do companies sell allergy-blocking supplements and promise that they will take away your fatigue? Because enough people are willing to buy them, plain and simple. The only thing lightened by these products is your wallet. My advice to those of you who think your fatigue comes from allergies is to ignore the pseudoscience, take your non-drowsy antihistamine when your nose swells to three times its normal size, and read on. The answer to your fatigue is still waiting to be discovered.

The Endocrine System

A seasoned medical school professor once told me, "All of life, from the dances of the ballerina to love's own waltz, boils down to two things: neurons that fire and glands that squirt." Though many people would take issue with this, the cold, biological facts probably aren't too far from the truth. From the embarrassingly amorous overtures of adolescent boys to the seismograph-sized mood swings of pregnancy, our hormones control more than we admit to—and more than we wish them to. They influence the way we think, the way we feel, and how we interact with others. Hormones also play a large role in governing the many functions of the body. We could call them the "Congress of Human Behavior." So, how do these glandular elixirs work?

To start with, let's note that hormones come from glands, and glands are what make up the endocrine system of which we speak. I'll also mention that the endocrine system contains more stewing chemicals than there are spices in a good cioppino recipe, and it boasts a complexity that few human disciplines can even imagine.

Nevertheless, I think that we can untangle this complicated web and elicit the causes of hormone-based fatigue. The number of common endocrine maladies are limited, and even the more rare conditions don't hide themselves in the bloodstream as some people think they do. Because of all the interacting substances in the endocrine system, a change in one level will affect something else; in other words, even when we can't see one chemical, we see its shadow. Your regular doctor should be able to diagnose for you the vast majority of endocrine-based conditions, and if she can't, an internist can. Endocrine specialists can also help guide you back to hormonal health. But before you start making phone calls and appointments, let's see if it's those glands of yours that are really causing your fatigue.

Thyroid disorders seem to be the most popular topic listed in both health journals and women's magazines, so I will begin with this misunderstood gland. Although I briefly discussed this back in Chapter Two, now I'm going to go into a lot more detail. The reason for this semi-rehashing? If I had a dime for every patient who walked into my office mistakenly convinced that their thyroid had gone awry and was causing them to gain weight and feel fatigued, I would be writing this book from a penthouse balcony in the Bahamas. I don't want you to be that misinformed patient. I want you to go to your doctor sounding like you know what you're talking about when you bring up hypothyroidism and other endocrine conditions that can cause fatigue.

Hypothyroidism, or low thyroid functioning, can occur for many reasons, the most common being from an attack by the immune system on the actual gland. This condition is called Hashimoto's thyroiditis. Other causes include surgical removal of the thyroid because of cancer, radiation treatments for an overactive thyroid, and pituitary failure, which we'll examine in just a minute. If you truly have hypothyroidism, your metabolism will drop and you'll have symptoms such as fatigue, hair loss (especially the outside third of the eyebrows, go figure), weight gain, constipation, slow heart rate, dry skin, and you'll feel cold all the time. Other disorders can produce some or all of these symptoms as well, however, which can fool you into believing that their thyroid has failed.

To find out if hypothyroidism (or another thyroid abnormality) is really your problem, a full thyroid profile (measuring TSH, T3, and T4) can be performed on your blood. TSH, or the thyroid-stimulating hormone, is a chemical released by the pituitary gland that prods the thyroid into making the hormones T3 and T4. T3 is the active hormone and makes up about twenty percent of the levels; T4 is inactive until converted into T3 in your body's tissues.

So now, let's look at pituitary failure. Like a thermostat that turns the furnace on when a house gets cold, the pituitary regulates the thyroid depending on the level of hormones in the bloodstream. In pituitary failure, TSH is low (because the pituitary gland can't make it) and T3 and T4 are low (because the thyroid isn't being told to make either hormone). This condition is somewhat rare, usually happening after the rapid blood loss that occurs during childbirth. Another cause of pituitary failure is an immune attack, wherein antibodies destroy the gland. I have seen only one case of this since starting my practice, and I have great interest in that patient, mostly because I am that patient. The disease destroyed my adrenal glands also. Thanks to an excellent physician, I lived to tell about it.

In most cases of hypothyroidism, though, pituitary failure is not the case. More often, your TSH will be high, and your pituitary will be begging your thyroid to make more hormones. T3 and T4 will be low because the thyroid, like most teenagers, just isn't listening. In mild hypothyroid cases—which are the majority of them—the TSH is slightly elevated, in the 5 to 15 range (normal being 0.5 to 5.5), and fatigue is generally not an issue.

The opposite problem, of course, is hyperthyroidism, an excess of thyroid hormones in your bloodstream. In this condition, the thyroid runs amuck and produces too much T3 and T4, or the doctor runs amuck and gives too much replacement hormone for your already—diagnosed hypothyroid problem. Either way, hyperthyroidism will give you a low TSH level, because the pituitary will have backed off its stimulation of the over-productive thyroid gland, and the T3 and T4 will be high. This state of elevated hormones can cause fatigue due to your body feeling like your foot is always on the gas pedal. Other symptoms of hyperthyroidism include problems cause by an elevated metabolism, such as sweating, rapid heart rate, and anxiety. Hyperthyroidism is treatable through surgery or radiation.

Before leaving the endocrine system, I need to discuss a few more topics, starting with the sex hormones. Let's face it, without them, life would just not be as interesting; tabloids would be wafer thin, and a bikini would only be a fashion statement. But as much fun as they can be when they course normally through your bloodstream, they can wreak havoc when they're unbalanced. Let's start with a look at estrogen. Yes, it's the woman hormone, but male readers, pay attention! Estrogen can cause problems for you, too—unless you think that fatigue, headache and prostatitis are normal, everyday occurrences and no cause for alarm whatsoever.

Three different estrogens—estrone, estradiol, and estriol—are found in the blood and tissues of the human body. In women, the ovaries and adrenal glands are the primary producers of these substances; in men, they come from the adrenals as well as through conversion from testosterone (the "You talkin' to me?" hormone) in the tissues by the enzyme aromatase. Estrogen must be balanced in both men and women by another hormone, progesterone, the body-made hormone that is the building block of many other hormones. Think of estrogen and progesterone as yin and yang, each needing the other for balance. One of the biggest reasons estrogen levels rise to excess is because of low progesterone, which at a diminished level cannot exert its lowering effect on the estrogen—it's a big, vicious circle. Whether you're menopausal or not, on hormones or not, or whether you're male or female, excess estrogen can cause a plethora of symptoms in your body, such as edema (unwanted swelling), depression, anxiety, obesity, loss of libido, and an increased risk of breast and prostate cancer. Short of a dozen tequila shooters and half as many bean burritos, no other chemical can make you feel so bad when it is in overabundance. It can be the reason people cling to their weight, the reason patients on antidepressants can't seem to get better, and the reason breast and prostate cancer are on the rise.

So, how and why do patients become excessive in their estrogen? We know that women on birth control pills and hormone replacement get that extra amount through these prescriptions. But what about everyone else, including the men? How do we become estrogen toxic, so to speak, especially those of us who don't take hormone supplements in any form? To put it simply, it can happen because of foods and progesterone deficiency, which comes predominantly from poor diet, stress, and low levels of exercise—kind of American culture in a nutshell, isn't it? There are also environmental toxins, to consider: Xenoestrogens, by-products of petroleum-based energy, raise estrogen levels, as do the steroids used to accelerate growth in poultry and livestock. Pesticides, like DDT, also drive those levels up and help create an imbalance of hormones.

So, what should you do if you feel like your estrogen and progesterone balance is off? What if you think that's what's causing your fatigue? Well, I recommend that you rule out all other causes of fatigue first. If you don't find any other reasonable cause, get some testing done Regular levels of estrogen and estrogen-stimulating hormones can be measured in your blood, and the xenoestrogens can be measure in saliva. Home saliva-testing kits are even being developed; check with a provider in your area.

On the other side of things, testosterone is made in both males and females and is responsible for bone strength, energy, muscle mass, libido, and the thrill you get from yelling, "Woo woo!" after imbibing excess alcohol. Deficiency of this hormone can affect your body's strength and structure, lower your libido, and diminish your vigor. Excessive levels of it in women can cause unwanted facial hair and other masculine features, and in men, it can make us act like ... well, men.

Testosterone levels can usually be measured easily in the bloodstream and most primary care practitioners can measure, diagnose, and treat abnormal levels in men or women. Failure to make testosterone in men happens usually because of testicular failure, which can occur at any age. In rarer cases, pituitary failure can lower the hormone's level. In women, failure usually occurs at menopause, from either biological shutdown or surgical removal of the ovaries.

Excess testosterone in men can result in men from over-supplementation (a fancy word for "taking too much," as in hormone pills), testicular tumors, or adrenal gland enlargement (hyperplasia). Women can get too much testosterone if they become overweight and resistant to their own insulin, which results in estrogen converting to testosterone in the body's fat. Fatigue can result from either excess or deficiency of testosterone, so your levels should be examined by your doctor if you're feeling fatigued and have the symptoms mentioned above.

DHEA is a chemical similar to testosterone that is produced by the adrenal glands in both men and women. It can convert to testosterone in both sexes and to estrogen in women. As we age, DHEA levels fall, reaching a low of about 20 percent of normal by the time we hit seventy. Originally, DHEA was just thought to be a building block of other hormones, but it's recently been discovered in the liver and kidney, making researchers believe that it may serve other functions. In one study, elderly patients with DHEA deficiencies were given daily supplements of 5 to 10 milligrams for women and 10 to 20 milligrams for men. Both sexes reported feeling more energy and stamina, with the women improving in 84 percent of cases, and the men improving 67 percent of the time. Because of the way DHEA converts to other hormones, make sure you and your doctor are very careful about over-supplementation; levels under 30 milligrams per day are considered very safe. And once again, I advise you to make sure that all other causes of fatigue are ruled out before testing your DHEA levels.

Cortisol is another adrenal hormone necessary for life, its function pivotal to the metabolism of the body's fat, protein, and carbohydrates. When cortisol levels drop, the pituitary calls out for more production of it with the hormone ACTH. When ACTH levels are elevated because the pituitary is trying very hard to stimulate sluggish adrenal glands, the excessive hormone stains the skin wherever it folds—for example, at the insides of your elbows or the backs of your knees. These darker streaks of skin are the hallmark of Addison's disease, a condition suffered by the late President Kennedy.

In pituitary failure, no ACTH can be made, so levels of both that and cortisol are low. Low cortisol levels can cause fatigue, low blood pressure, muscle aches, and depression. Most cases of this occur after rapid discontinuation of medical steroids. In most instances, the adrenals can be coaxed back to normal production again, but autoimmune diseases can render the pituitary, adrenal, or both as worthless as a campaign promise, causing the adrenal glands to fail. Patients with permanent shutdown will need to take steroid pills regularly the rest of their lives.

The best time to measure levels of cortisol is in the morning, after an overnight fast. Any primary care provider can order this test. If a blood test is low or borderline, or your caregiver is unsure of your adrenal status, a corticotropin stimulation test can be ordered. In this study, ACTH (corticotropin) is given and blood is drawn every half an hour for three hours or so to see if the adrenal glands respond. ACTH is what your pituitary gland secretes to turn on your adrenal glands.

Some doctors have experimentally administered steroids (a product of adrenal glands) to see if they will make a patient with low cortisol levels feel better. However, this can be quite dangerous, due to the side effects that unneeded cortisone can bring to the body. Excessive cortisol production, or taking excessive amounts of pills or shots (as mentioned above), can also cause fatigue. If this is the case, the face usually becomes fat (called "moon face") and the back of the neck can layer with fat, producing what doctors call the "buffalo hump." Patients with thick fat deposits from poor diet have crossed my path more than once, and I have checked their cortisol level to make sure that it was normal. Thankfully, excessive cortisol in the body is a rare condition—it's actually called Cushing's Syndrome—and it isn't a common cause of fatigue.

"Okay," you're saying. "I've just about had it with the Endocrine system. No more glands, please!" Believe me, I understand, it's not really the most fascinating of subjects. But I only have one more hormone to discuss, and it is the most important one—in fact, it will the most important thing I have discussed in this book so far. It's called insulin, and I'm going to go ahead and say that it is indeed this section's "gland finale."

Insulin is the taxicab that carries sugar to the muscle cells for storage. A low insulin level allows glucose (that's sugar) to build up in the bloodstream, causing Diabetes. Blurry vision, excessive urination, and thirst, combined with your fatigue, could be signs of diabetes. If you have these symptoms, seek medical help immediately; once your sugar level is normalized, you should feel a whole lot better.

Although Diabetes is critical, and tested for at virtually every physical, insulin usually comes up during discussions of fatigue because of the excesses of it that commonly occur in both men and women. Besides making us fat, triggering occasional low sugar episodes, and lowering our metabolisms, high levels of insulin make us tired—real tired! Excessive insulin comes not from pancreas problems (it is secreted by the pancreas in the first place), but from insulin resistance. What this means is that when target cells in the muscle—those are the cells that insulin sticks the sugar into—become insensitive or resistant to insulin, they'll refuse to store the sugar, and so sugar levels in the body will begin to rise. The body recognizes this increase and kicks out more insulin, hoping to find enough target cells to accept the sugar. The result is high levels of insulin in the blood, a tired pancreas, and a very tired patient who might also have the added bonus of a weight-gain problem.

So, why do we become insulin resistant? There are three main reasons. First, insulin has a genetic component. Patients with a strong family history of Diabetes have a higher risk of insulin resistance than those who do not. Second, our modern culture doesn't promote exercise or anything that resembles it—we don't have to hunt our own food or even raise our own garage doors by hand anymore. This lack of consistent, continuous exercise makes the doors on our target muscle cells harder to open. And to make things worse, the more weight gain the resistance causes, the more resistance is caused and of course, vice versa. As we get more and more resistant from our increased weight, our pancreas kicks out more and more insulin. This snowball effect not only tips the weight scales higher and drives us towards Diabetes, it also makes us fatigued.

Patients with this condition have many things in common, including high insulin levels in the blood (especially when drawn first thing in the morning), obesity, and elevated fats (cholesterol and triglycerides) in their bloodstreams. Doctors call this phenomenon Metabolic Syndrome. The health problems that this condition causes, from heart disease to weight gain, are second only to the weariness it produces.

So, what causes the fatigue? Besides the free fall of neurotransmitters (brain chemicals) caused by the aversion to exercise and the universal gravitational attraction to the couch, the hormone insulin has a strong fatiguing effect on the body. The tiredness peaks after meals that are rich in carbohydrates, which break down into sugar. Recently, my doctor performed an insulin stress test on me, wherein he dripped insulin into my vein to drive down my sugar and test my adrenal glands. Talk about fatigue—I felt so weak that my 105-pound wife could have arm-wrestled me and won. During the test, I needed help sliding back up in bed, the weakness was so intense. Trust me, insulin fatigues us all, and the carbohydrate-rich diet that Americans usually eat can push our levels to six times the normal on any given day. With 40 percent of the population being "insulin resistant," this creates a lot of post-prandial fatigue (that means it happens after you eat). In some patients, the insulin levels never drop, and the weariness lasts all day.

How can you shake this condition? More will be said about that at the end of this book, but for now, let's think about the actual problem. If sugar cannot be placed into the muscle cell because it is resistant, then we should avoid ... that's right, SUGAR! And sugar comes in many forms, all of which are products of carbohydrate breakdown. By limiting the quantity of carbohydrates (a.k.a. starches) that we consume, we will limit the amount of sugar that has to be stored. And if we limit our amount of sugar, our insulin levels will drop. The decrease in insulin will then stop the drain of energy, not to mention the drag on the metabolism. Because not all starches are created equal, it's important to know which ones are the best to eat. Though I won't tread deeply into this right now, rule number one regarding carbohydrates states, "If the starch is white—such as potatoes, rice, or bread—don't eat it."

The second rule is as simple as the first. If your lack of exercise is what's causing you to be resistant to insulin, you can fix this situation by—yes, you guessed it, exercising! With continuous movement, the cell walls of the muscle become more accepting to sugar, and the levels of needed insulin drop. With less insulin in the bloodstream, the body is less fatigued. Use these diet and exercise tips, and your energy levels should return to normal.

So, there, we've done it! Together, we have walked our way through practically all of the living body to find the various physiologic causes of fatigue. We have only one main section to go—a chapter where most of you will find the roots of your weariness. No, it's not the "soul system," and you don't have to mail me 10 percent of your income. It's the complex inner workings of the neurotransmitters, found between your ears, that causes the majority of fatigue. Low levels of these brain chemicals produces more fatigue than everything else that I have covered to this point!

But before I launch into that discussion, I have one more thing to clear up. The subject is Chronic Fatigue, an illness that is terribly over-diagnosed and poorly understood. For those of you who carry this diagnosis, please read this section before moving on. It is critical to find out if you were properly diagnosed. And for those of you who don't have this diagnosis, well ... don't skip ahead. You should read this section too.

GET A HANDLE ON
CHRONIC FATIGUE SYNDROME

Perhaps the only thing more confusing than the diagnosis of Chronic Fatigue Syndrome (CFS) is the American Tax Code. The diagnosis of CFS is fraught with disaster, not because the condition is so confusing, but because many clinicians stick this label on patients incorrectly. I would love to tell you that doctors are correct in their diagnoses all the time, but we're human too, despite the years of education; sometimes, we're just as fallible as the next guy.

CFS is a specific diagnosis, not a general category of tired people. I would be willing to bet that for every ten patients with this diagnosis, only one or two actually meet the criteria for the disease. Why would I make a statement like that? Because I see patient after tired patient, most with curable causes of fatigue, coming into my office with incorrect CFS diagnoses. Many have suffered for a long time, needlessly in most cases. I want to set the record straight so that those with true CFS can be treated appropriately, and those who don't have it can find the real cause of their tiredness.

For a proper definition of CFS, you could access a variety of sources. One typical source, which is not always the best, is the World Wide Web. Although the Internet is a virtual galaxy of information, not all of it is accurate. In fact, to start your own medical Web site, you need only two things: a computer and fingers to type. Any person could run his own medical information page and get ten thousand hits a day—while also getting a D average in biology. My point is this: getting on the Internet to solve your medical problem is like typing "religion" into a search engine to find meaning and purpose in your life. So let's look instead to the medical texts to learn more about CFS.

Many patients have fatigue that has become chronic (lasting longer than six weeks). But for an acceptable diagnosis of CFS, you need to be have suffered for at least three weeks with sore throat, fever, and swollen lymph glands, just prior to the beginning of the fatigue. This viral-like illness must precede the long-term exhaustion or a CFS diagnosis cannot be made. This is where the majority of patients get their misdiagnosis.

The fatigue associated with CFS generally abates within five years, and in most cases, two years. It is christened with the above viral-like symptoms and is undoubtedly an immune-related syndrome. Though scientists don't know exactly what causes it, there are some general treatments that can be applied. Finding out that your long-term tiredness is not CFS is very important, because a correct diagnosis can follow, along with the appropriate therapy. Those of you with CFS do have some hope, along with some treatment options. I will try to summarize what we know and don't know about CFS and offer some suggestions on how to combat its fatigue.

Originally, CFS was erroneously linked to the Epstein-Barr virus, the nasty little pathogen responsible for mononucleosis. Because of the way mononucleosis fatigues its victim and because of its initial symptoms, this was a reasonable assumption. But after blood studies were done on tens of thousands of people, it became apparent that many with CFS had no evidence of infection with the Epstein-Barr virus, and many with the antibodies for Epstein-Barr didn't have CFS. Before the results of these studies reached the eyes and ears of primary care practitioners, however, labs all over the country were running Epstein-Barr tests, and multitudes of frustrated individuals were roaming the earth with Epstein-Barr neon signs flickering on their foreheads. Epstein-Barr became the new excuse for lying around on the couch eating chips and watching cable TV all day.

The sadness in all of this was that some of the healthcare professionals either didn't get the memo or failed to communicate it to their supposed Epstein-Barr patients. More than ten years after the Centers for Disease Control and the College of Infectious Disease declared Epstein-Barr not to be the cause of CFS, an unbelievable number of people come to my office with those neon signs still flickering over their brows. Often, I diagnose their true cause of fatigue and they do get well.

So, if Epstein-Barr isn't the cause of CFS, what is? If I knew for sure, I would be living in the islands and sipping a foo-foo drink at this moment, instead of working for a living. No one really knows for sure, but best bets indicate that CFS is caused by something that kicks the body's immune system in the proverbial groin and leaves it floundering in fatigue. For a while, it was rumored that cytomegalavirus, the other cause of mononucleosis, might be the culprit. But that idea was quickly dispelled.

Reasonable theories from the Center for Disease Control, who provides the most reliable information regarding CFS, are limited to four. First is the immune system dysfunction theory, which I mentioned above. A second theory, and the one which is most promising, revolves around immune-related cells called cytokines. A study in which cytokines were injected into normal, non-fatigued patients showed that fatigue could be induced with this substance. One discrepancy in that theory hails from another study, which showed high levels of cytokines measured in patients who had already recovered from CFS. What does this mean? Perhaps the body learns to turn off the fatiguing effect of these cytokines to beat the disease. Or perhaps these substances have nothing to do with CFS; hopefully, time will tell on that one. Other theories regarding immune deregulation are also being looked at, but none is more promising at this time than the cytokine theory.

A third theory asserts that CFS is caused by naturally mediated hypotension, a condition that causes chronically low blood pressure and pulse rates. The validity of this theory is bolstered by the fact that CFS patients have a positive tilt test four times more often than they do a negative test; the tilt test involves checking for a decline in blood pressure and pulse when a patient is tilted seventy degrees on a moveable table. Some CFS sufferers have improved with Florinef, a pill that helps the body retain salt and raises the blood pressure. A trial is currently underway to see if this chemical will help CFS patients. I'm not a proponent of this theory, seeing how some of my CFS patients have hypertension—high blood pressure, obviously the opposite of hypotension—and I have to give them medicine to reduce it. Perhaps the hypotension arises from the depression that comes frequently with CFS; depressive moods can in fact cause a positive tilt test.

A fourth plausible cause of CFS is the suppression of the HPA axis, which is comprised of the glands that support cortisol production in the body. Normally, as mentioned prior, the pituitary gland in the brain tells the adrenal gland (which sits on the kidney) to make this hormone, and then the pituitary gland monitors that production. This hypothesis seems weak, considering that cortisone shots don't seem to help most CFS patients. Also, the patients don't have symptoms or blood-work reflective of Addison's disease (remember, that means low cortisol). Despite this fact, enough concern exists that trials and research on this theory are still underway.

The last theory of CFS to be discussed is really not a theory at all, but a scam that the CDC exposes on its Web site. Along with just about every medical text that weighs down my bookshelves, the CDC site states fairly clearly that no vitamin-herb-mineral deficiency is at the root of this energy-choking illness. Any person trying to sell a CFS patient an "all natural" panacea is just plain stealing from them. Don't waste your money on any supplement, other than a cheap multivitamin. Anything else is just a waste of money.

So, how do CFS patients find relief for their exhaustion? Well, remember that the prescription for health may be different for each person. Experimentation with any combination of the following ideas may produce the right balance for you.

CFS treatment begins, very simply, with good nutrition. The CDC, along with most experts, teaches that no return to health, be it from cancer or CFS, can be fueled with garbage. Fruits, vegetables, and complex carbohydrates are the building blocks of mitochondria, the part of the body's cells responsible for energy. Potato chips, ice cream, and fast food are fuel for high insulin levels and disaster. A dietician or your primary care provider can give you more information on this.

The second cornerstone of treatment for CFS is a regular amount of light exercise. The key word here is light, because not knowing when to stop can lead you to an energy crunch the following day. Walking, pool therapy, and light biking seem to be the best. Whatever you decide to try, make sure that you enjoy it and that you don't overdo it. Over time, you will learn the right amount of activity.

Another treatment is cognitive therapy, which works surprisingly well in addition to other treatments. A therapist trained in this area of psychology can help unlock the energy to which your mind holds the key. Fatigue can be a learned activity, and can become rather expected by your body. Cognitive therapy can help overcome this stinkin' thinkin' and unleash some energy for you. Multiple studies have shown that it works.

One critical therapy in the treatment of CFS is antidepressant treatment, even for those of you who don't feel depressed! The reason I propose this is that all chronic illnesses, regardless of type, deplete one or more neurotransmitters in the brain (serotonin, norepinephrine, and dopamine.) SSRI medications, such as Prozac, affect the levels of serotonin in your brain, and SNRI's, such as Effexor or Cymbalta, deal with the serotonin and norepinephrine; all these medications help raise the levels of these neurotransmitters and can increase your energy. Dopamine, the third neurotransmitter that is known to be related to fatigue, can be elevated with Wellbutrin, another pharmaceutical pill. Interestingly, smokers seem to do best with this drug because nicotine is known to temporarily elevate dopamine. Each of these prescriptions can be safely combined with each other to produce maximum energy.

Depressed mood is only one symptom of actual clinical depression, wherein fatigue and sleep irregularities are much more common complaints. The type of depression we're talking about here is not sadness about your condition, but rather a chemical deficiency caused by a chronic disease. If your level of neurotransmitters gets low enough, a deflated mood can set in. Most of my CFS patients have a normal mood, but suffer many of the other symptoms of low neurotransmitters, such as fatigue, decreased concentration, appetite irregularities, and sleep disturbance. I will talk more deeply regarding this chemistry in the next chapter.

Before we leave CFS and delve into the number one reason people in America are fatigued, I want to list some of the experimental treatments that show some promise in CFS therapy. When you've tried the above-mentioned therapies and you're not adequately improved, it is reasonable to experiment with unproven treatments, if they are safe and have some science behind them. Bogus therapies, such as high colonics (colon washing), are more masochistic than medicinal and should be avoided. We know that toxins in the colon don't cause the fatigue of CFS, because many who have their colons removed due to other diseases still develop CFS later in life. I would recommend sticking to one of the therapies listed below.

One of the most promising medicines worth trying is a new drug for narcolepsy (chronic daytime sleepiness—we looked at that in the last chapter) called Provigil. This chemical is a non-stimulant that can help you stay vibrant throughout the day. Side effects are fairly low and include possible dry mouth, insomnia and tremor, but most patients tolerate it fairly well. The only problem I have had using this medication is getting insurance companies to pay for it; at $200 per month, it can get expensive. Sometimes it helps if a specialist lobbies the insurers on your behalf, so if you have a problem getting your insurance to pay for your prescription, talk to the doctor who prescribed it to you. Maybe she can help.

Ampligen, a stimulator of interferon (a protein that inhibits virus development in the body), is another experimental medication for CFS. Currently undergoing trials, it is not approved for use yet, but it holds some promise for CFS patients. As with other drugs, use of Ampligen would require monitoring your liver functioning with blood tests, as the drug could cause a toxic build up in the organ. Time will tell if this product will be helpful.

Gamma-globulin, another active immune system component, has been mentioned as a possible therapy. Owing to the immune-related theory of the disease, it seems reasonable to think this might help. Early trials have been somewhat disappointing, but work continues to be done by those who espouse this theory.

Short-term steroids have also been tried, but side effects can become a problem if a you take them for long periods of time. Short bursts of cortisone also sometimes give temporary relief to some CFS sufferers; this treatment is based on the HPA axis theory mentioned earlier. However, I personally have found only a handful of people who have received a positive result from this.

DHEA also holds some promise in treating CFS. As aforementioned, it is a building block of testosterone, but has been found in other parts of the body besides those that usually accept the sex steroids. This has made some scientists suspect that there are other roles for DHEA and that a trial of this non-prescription medicine might be helpful beyond the sexual arena. I recommend that DHEA levels be drawn first, though many of my patients find that just an over-the-counter supplement works well for them.

On the negative side, I want to mention two experimental treatments that you probably should avoid. One is Ketapressin, a medicine made from pig livers. It is ineffective and has too high a risk factor; it has been tied to some fairly serious allergic reactions. Second is colonic washing, which has shown no promise of helping anyone. Remember ... where there is desperation, within two feet stands a salesman. So, please, be careful when choosing treatment for your CFS. If it sounds too good to be true, it probably is.

As I close the chapter on CFS, I want you to realize the complexity of this disease. Many people think they have the answer to CFS, but in many cases, it just may not be so. In general, follow a routine of good nutrition and gentle exercise. Add in a positive-energy neurotransmitter agent such as Prozac, Effexor, or Wellbutrin. If none of these three drugs help, move on to the experimental agents listed above. Mix in some cognitive therapy, finish the rest of this book, learn more about what's ailing you, and whatever you do—never, ever give up.

LEARN ABOUT FATIGUE'S NUMBER ONE CAUSE

Okay, cheaters. For those of you who have skipped ahead to this chapter, get back to the beginning of the book. There's a lot of information there that I promise you will need to know. For those of you hard workers turning onto this chapter from the last, congratulations and welcome.

Twelve years and at least seventy-five hundred complaints of fatigue into my medical career, I have finally learned something: few health professionals are interested in treating fatigue. The doctors that my fatigued patients frequented before coming to me usually performed appropriate blood work, and for the most part, proper testing ruled out the bad diseases such as cancer and anemia. But after a pat on the back and a reassurance that nothing was wrong, the patients were turned loose to struggle with their own fatigue. Many who sought out new practitioners or second opinions were often given the same line: "There is nothing I can do for you."

How could so many doctors be so clueless? What could possibly cause such weariness in so many people, contribute to such morbidity, and yet evade the scrutinizing gaze of so many professionals? And what is the number one cause of fatigue? I'll dispense with the suspense and reply to the question directly.

The answer is deep in the gray matter of the brain. It is essentially an unmeasurable entity—meaning that it can't be found in the blood—and it is the driving force of our existence. Our motivation, energy, focus, and short-term memory originate at this spot. So does our ability to fall asleep, stay asleep, and wake up rested. In addition, appetite, mood, patience, and concentration arise from this part of the body.

This section of our brain, responsible for the above functions, is the place where the neurotransmitters interact and assist the neurons in communication. It is the number one place where fatigue arises. Because these chemicals can't be measured or quantified, it is often overlooked in the cause for patient's weariness. So, how does this system work ... and more importantly, how do we find out if our problems are born out of neurotransmitter turmoil?

Neurotransmitters Explained

Four major neurotransmitters, plus a few minor ones, keep modern man moving, thinking, acting, and feeling in response to and in interaction with his environment. The intricacy of this complex, communicating group of chemicals never ceases to amaze the scientists who pry open the secrets of the brain. In three one-thousandths of a second, neurons, the basic cells of our brain and nervous system, transmit electrical and chemical information to other neurons in the brain. This interaction brings about conscious thought.

Billions of times per second this happens, in trillions upon trillions of different patterns—giving us our individuality, quirks, gifts, and even life itself. From the inspiring sounds of a soothing symphony to the calculations that allow a rocket to lift gracefully from its launch pad, the firing of neurotransmitters allows us to think, feel, and act—sometimes reflecting back the image of a Maker and sometimes projecting the callous instincts of the wild.

Four major neurotransmitters run this engine of our being, one for physical movement and three for the movement of our minds. The former, acetacholine, is a topic for neurology and not really relevant to our current topic. The latter, however, are central elements in the analysis of fatigue. Their unique function is to motivate the movement of the muscles, but not to move them, and to fuel the pistons of the mind.

The three neurotransmitters responsible for our energy levels, amongst many other things, are serotonin, norepinephrine, and dopamine—you may remember their names from the last chapter, when we looked at medications used to control them. If we wish to comprehend what has happened to our mojo, so to speak, we must first understand these three chemicals and how they work. For those readers whose knowledge of chemistry is limited to what happens between the sheets, take heart—I will keep it simple. The more you learn about how your body works, the better chance you have in tracking down the cause of your maladies.

Serotonin, probably the best known of the triad, is responsible for our impulses, irritability, anxiety, mood, and emotions, along with sex drive, appetite, and energy. Norepinephrine is responsible for anxiety, energy, and mood also. In addition, we find it supporting our ability to block pain, our self-control, and interest in the world outside us. The third neurotransmitter, dopamine, is responsible for our motivation, energy, sex drive, and appetite. As you can see, there is a lot of overlap and shared responsibility. And because energy, or lack thereof, can be found in all three neurotransmitters (or even in a combination of the three), I would like to explore each in more detail.

All neurotransmitters are chemical communicators that function by firing off the neurons they're next to, sparking communication the way a conversation might erupt if you bumped into an old friend at the supermarket. When this dialogue spreads across imprinted, or previously used, pathways of the brain, certain tasks are accomplished—such as calculating how much debt you are in after paying your taxes, feeling the blistering burn of anger after an eighteen wheeler cuts you off, or daydreaming during the Reverend Dogooder's sermon. Trillions of links between hundreds of billions of neurons all fire in well-orchestrated concert to produce consciousness, beliefs, and pursuit of dreams. Though genetics, nature, and different life experiences shape these pathways and make us all different, we really have a lot in common with one another.

After a neuron has released the proper neurotransmitter and it strikes a receptor on another cell, the neurotransmitter is broken down by an enzyme (monoamine oxidase) and the pieces are recycled later. The enzyme performs this "re-uptake," or recycling of the neurotransmitter, quickly, and all of the chunks are taken back to the neuron.

In the brain as a whole, at any given moment, a certain quantity of neurotransmitters exists, both in an active state and a certain amount in pieces. Fatigue occurs when certain neurotransmitters are broken down too quickly, and the level of the whole, usable ones are less than normal. Depending on what transmitters are missing, and where, symptoms such as dizziness, low concentration, loss of sex drive, or memory loss may accompany the fatigue.

To make things a little more complex, let's add in that there are about twenty kinds of each of the three different neurotransmitters, each with a slightly different role. Depending on which of the sixty or so substances are in shorter supply in your brain, you could display a wide variety of symptoms, with or without fatigue. Deficiencies of these chemicals occur for a variety of reasons, which we'll get into in a minute or two.

First, I want to address the fact that you may be wrinkling your brow and thinking, "I'm not depressed. What on earth is he telling me this for?"

And I will tell you that I know you're not depressed—but I also know that this information can still apply to you. Neurotransmitters may cause depression or anxiety in some people, but for every one person whose levels have slipped down that low, twenty or more have milder symptoms, up to and including our old friend fatigue. Energy seems to be one of the first pieces of cargo that the brain throws overboard when it begins to flounder. At first it may be just a mild fatigue at the end of the day, but if the problem is ignored, it can escalate into a more serious fatigue that sends nice folks to their medical provider, searching for an answer.

So, how do we find a neurotransmitter deficiency? PET (positive emission topography) scanners can find them, but, unfortunately, they are extremely expensive, usually available only in a few research centers, and usually not covered by insurance. Plus, the average Joe can't just walk in and get scanned, though it would make my job easier if they could. Because of these obstacles to having a PET done, we doctors often try to rule out any other causes of fatigue to see if the symptoms fit neurotransmitter loss.

What causes a person to have low neurotransmitters, anyway? It might be easier to answer the question, "What doesn't lower our neurotransmitters?" There are a host of conditions that deplete our energy chemicals, and the task of reviewing each one may be a bit daunting. But like the medical cases of fatigue, every perpetrator can be identified, clarified, and classified. Let's try to do a little bit of that ourselves right now.

Essentially, anything that stimulates monoamine oxidase (the chemical that breaks down the neurotransmitters) can cause fatigue. Some of the factors listed below give good explanations for how this enzyme is turned off and on, and some don't. In many cases, we just have to rely on clinical experience to tie activities or conditions with lowered neurotransmitters. In some instances—actually, in most instances—more than one culprit is to blame. Let's take a look at each and see if we can spot the things that might be stealing your thunder.

Factors That Affect—What Could Be Lowering Your Neurotransmitters?

Genetics

An estimated 30 percent of all people have a genetic defect that will cause low levels of neurotransmitters at some point in their lives. As with other inherited diseases, some of these chromosomal abnormalities are strongly expressed—the person gets a more severe case of the unwanted condition—or mildly expressed—the person may suffer only limited symptoms of the disease. Defects can occur with any of the three neurotransmitters or they can occur in combination. The sixty-plus collective subtypes of serotonin, norepinephrine and dopamine all can cause fatigue when they drop below normal levels.

Diseases that people suffer may clue us in to which of their neurotransmitters might be in short supply. Fibromyalgia seems to lower both serotonin and norepinephrine, while migraine and irritable bowel patients, along with those that suffer from anxiety and/or panic attacks, usually have pure serotonin deficiency. Marathon runners and people addicted to pornography nicotine, drugs, gambling, and the like, usually suffer from low dopamine levels. It should be mentioned that just because a person has a genetic defect, doesn't mean he is destined to get the disease. New genetic research tells us that stressors in the environment can turn these genes on and bring on the condition, the way poor diet might bring on Diabetes in someone with the condition in his family.

These generalities are just that—generalities—but they can help guide you and your doctor when choosing proper treatment. It is hoped that genetic testing can help assess your DNA and help your doctors prescribe treatments more accurately, but really, treatments often rely on educated guesses.

Chronic Illness

Chronic diseases weigh on our neurotransmitters like ninety-year-old pensioners on the payroll of a mom-and-pop business. From asthma to high blood pressure, illnesses that hang around drag down our energy by putting a chronic strain on our neurotransmitters. No one is exactly sure why or how this happens, but it's been documented a thousand times over. Whether it is the worry that comes with a disabling condition, or more likely, an unknown pathway that siphons off the proper brain compounds, long term conditions seem to impose themselves on our neurotransmitters and induce a disabling, or just a distracting fatigue. Recommendations on how to manage our neurochemicals in the face of these diseases will be discussed later.

Pain

Although chronic pain certainly would fit in the category of chronic illness, I wanted this nagging, long-term discomfort to land in its own spotlight. When a person lives in continuous hurt, be it ongoing back pain or sickle cell anemia, neurotransmitter depletion is the rule, not the exception. People with chronic pain develop chemical abnormalities in virtually every case. These are the unforgiving laws of chemistry that don't obey our wishes, wants, or personal strengths. And what makes chronic pain so detestable is that the very neurotransmitters that it depletes, we must use to lessen ordinary pain signals. It's a vicious circle that destroys the very thing we need to reduce the pain. Thus, it is important to manage the disease of pain appropriately, following the advice of a certified pain clinic.

Vascular Disease

There is something magical—no, more like diabolical—about vascular illness. Blockage of any artery or the resulting lack of oxygen, be it from heart attack or stroke, lowers the levels of neurotransmitters and produces a tremendous fatigue. Even patients who have had surgery on their hearts or arteries often find themselves tired shortly thereafter. Frequently, they seek out cardiologists to solve this riddle of lost energy, but after their tests come back normal, they're left to flounder in rehab programs, trying to get their energy levels back, completely unaware of the neurotransmitter connection.

An estimated 70 percent of people with vascular illness suffer fatigue because of lowered neurotransmitters. The mechanism of the resultant fatigue is unknown, though it has been shown to have nothing to do with the person's mental state; that is, she isn't depressed over her condition. Many of these people feel better physically after the restoration of blood flow to the heart or brain, yet end up exhausted due to the loss of neurotransmitters. If the condition isn't diagnosed correctly, or if it doesn't fix itself, the person can slip further down the neurochemical slide and confront a major depression. I mention this for a variety of reasons, the most important being a study that showed that lack of treatment of neurotransmitter deficiency in such vascular cases increases mortality significantly. In other words, people die from the combination of their vascular problems and the untreated chemical imbalance. So, if you know someone who has undergone any type of vascular procedure, suffered a heart attack or stroke, and has struggled with fatigue ever since, please enlighten them about neurotransmitters and encourage them to seek treatment. A reduction in their life expectancy hangs in the balance.

Fibromyalgia

We've already looked at this chronically disabling condition already, but I'm going to mention it again, because fibromyalgia can cause—or perhaps, may be caused by—low neurotransmitters. It is the "chicken or the egg" concept, but I can attest that it is almost impossible to treat fibromyalgia without medicines that augment the neurotransmitters. For more information on this disease, please see the "Rheumatologic System" section in Chapter Four.

Psychiatric Illness

Perhaps it seems a bit obvious that mental disorders cause low levels of neurotransmitters; it's like saying that a link has been found between college parties and alcohol consumption. But these illnesses, specifically bipolar disorder and ADHD, are chronic manipulators of neurotransmitters. These diseases can fill you with superhuman power in one breath, and in the next, leave you drowning in a sea of fatigue.

Bipolar disorder is very good at hiding from accurate diagnosis. Where major depression can allow a person to slip slowly into a disabling fatigue, bipolar disorder (also known as manic depression) plunges the unsuspecting sufferer from highs to lows without warning. The patient might have six straight months of "good days," but could then crash land into a two-month sabbatical in bed, often without warning or explanation. It is estimated that 30 percent or more of people who are under medical care for anxiety or depression really have undiagnosed bipolar disorder. This is important because the traditional agents used to treat milder conditions, the standard antidepressants, can actually trigger the roller coaster ups and downs of bipolar disorder. So with antidepressants being prescribed at record rates in America and Europe, this can be of great concern. And because it takes an average of ten years to identify a bipolar patient, many people suffer the highs and lows because of improper treatment with typical antidepressants.

For all of you who think you don't have bipolar disorder, think again. More than a million have gone undiagnosed, suffering from the whimsical swings of their neurotransmitters. Clues to the possibility that you may have bipolar disorder include a family history of manic depression or hospitalization of close relatives with "nervous breakdowns," and periods in your life where a lot of sleep could be lost and not really be missed.

Anyone with this condition can experience highs and lows in their energy cycle, but some never get the luxury of the high and continually live in the basement. Medications may offer some short relief, but rarely does it last more than two weeks, and sometimes, they may even make the bipolar person worse. For this small subset of people, both the diagnosed and the undiagnosed, controlling the mood is a must before trying to lift the energy.

If the term bipolar scares you, please don't let it. To see if you are bipolar, even mildly, log onto Lilly.com and take the online screening test. If you score positive for bipolar, or score even borderline, print out your answer sheet and talk to your family practitioner or a psychiatrist to see if you can find professional assistance. Remember, at least two thirds of patients aren't diagnosed—and actually, it's probably more than that.

Another misdiagnosed psychiatric illness, well known for its erratic bouncing between energy and fatigue, is ADHD. Once thought to be a disorder of children only, specialists now tell us that two-thirds of cases persist into adulthood. People with ADHD can have periods of fluctuating energy and motivation, mood swings, difficulty concentrating, restlessness, and trouble following instructions. Often, despite their symptoms, they able to function and thrive in top professions,, but suffer in other aspects of their lives.

It is sometimes hard to tell bipolar illness and ADHD apart, but a difference can be drawn from looking at how persistent the disease is. Where ADHD arises from childhood, bipolar disorder starts later in life and, as previously mentioned, comes and goes. In many cases, people with ADHD never experience the "highs" that some bipolar people feel and only have periods of exhaustion; either way, if you have any kind of fluctuant moods along with your fatigue, seek professional help. To be screened for either condition, go to Lilly.com for a diagnostic questionnaire, or see a good psychiatrist.

Major Depression

Major depression is easier to diagnose than the above illnesses, yet the majority of patients with low energy don't know or believe that they are depressed. The sadness that people generally associate with depression is only one of fifteen symptoms of the disorder. Sleep abnormalities, appetite fluctuations, fatigue, dizziness, loss of short-term memory, concentration problems, anhedonia (lowered zeal for life), and emotional ups and downs are just some of the other symptoms. Not everyone experiences the same set of symptoms, and as mentioned previously, dysfunction progresses slowly with depression. The decline is gradual and can go unnoticed. One day you can wake up and wonder, "When did I start feeling this way?" If you have the symptoms listed above, see your primary care provider or a good psychologist for advice on how to pull yourself out of your depressed state.

Dysthymia

For those of you who have plodded through this book saying, "That's not me, that's not me," and who are probably wondering if your money would have been better spent on a bag of coffee beans, hang on, because this could be it. This topic will be where the cause of most cases of fatigue will be found.

Dysthymia is a neurotransmitter problem similar to depression, but not exactly the same. It is a condition wherein changes in certain chemicals cause fatigue; unlike genetic deficiencies that produce the plethora of symptoms, dysthymia can give you a disabling fatigue and no other symptoms. In many cases, your mood can be normal for the most part, but your drive and energy are lacking. It is a tiring condition that has risen dramatically in post-9/11 America.

People with dysthymia (some may actually call it a very mild depression) hoist themselves out of the sack and go to work every day—just so that they can pay their bills and buy another set of sheets for the bed that they long to be back in as soon as possible. With the loss of energy comes a frequent drop in motivation and chronic physical complaints; because neurotransmitters reduce pain signals as part of their job, their absence in a person with dysthymia can cause a laundry list of general aches and pains. As a result of this, they may go for a physical exam, but they will usually find no diseases that could explain the fatigue that they're feeling.

Although the cause of dysthymia is sometimes genetic, exogenous (external world) factors play a greater role—especially stress. Keeping up with the Jones's, longer work hours, soccer practice for three different kids, and a host of additional sub-conscious stresses have all chained us to the hamster wheel. We are all aware of the weights that hang around our necks, such as finances, and shelter. We worry about terrorism, in our own country and abroad. We have teleological issues—where did I come from, and where am I going?—and worries about our family's health and wellbeing. To me, it is obvious that in our attempts to reconcile the spiritual, physical, mental, and social realms in which we live, we frequently ask too much of ourselves and get overwhelmed. The resultant neurotransmitter deficiency drives our fatigue and steals our energy. This produces the vast majority of fatigue that I see from day to day.

Seasonal Affective Disorder

If you live in the northern climate and find your energy levels falling just about the time that the sun runs away from us each fall, consider seasonal affective disorder as the pillager of your potency. This condition is similar to dysthymia and results from a lack of sunlight absorbed through the eyes as the days get shorter. The pineal gland, a tiny piece of your brain, converts sunlight to serotonin. If there is a lack of sun stimulation, serotonin levels drop, and a dysthymia—like fatigue sets in. In more severe cases, actual depression develops.

The key to unlocking this diagnosis lies in the time that the low energy strikes. Problems during days with shorter sunlight periods would lead us towards seasonal affective disorder as a diagnosis. Yearlong problems, without the cyclical pattern, point to dysthymia. Your primary care practitioner can help you narrow down the culprit, but for now, let's move on and find out how to get back your neurotransmitters, your energy, or both.

CHAPTER SEVEN

FIND YOUR FIRE

The treatment of fatigue is based on the demon that drives it. The medical poultice that we use is matched to the pathological spell that has been cast. In other words, once your cause of fatigue has been discovered, the appropriate treatment can then be applied. For those tired people who are not sure of their diagnosis, don't worry; Chapter Eight will help you, along with your doctor, dredge out your diagnosis.

As I was saying, then, treatment is diagnosis-specific. If thyroid disease is the cause of your fatigue, thyroid medication is the appropriate therapy. If anemia is the perpetrator, iron therapy would be more appropriate, along with an investigation into the cause of the anemia. I'm sure you get the picture.

But for those of you whose fatigue comes from a neurotransmitter deficiency—and I predict that's over 90 percent of you—I will expound on the medicinal and non-medicinal ways of raising your brain chemical levels and bringing back the old you. In most cases, there isn't just one answer; a combination of therapies is often the safest and most prudent route back to good health.

Regardless of the cause of neurochemical poverty, be it a slow decline due to bad genes or just layer upon layer of stress, many pathways of treatment are available. And let me say something at this juncture if I haven't conveyed it already: Every person has the right to feel good, be energetic, and feel a zeal for life! My aim is to let those of you who suffer know that you should not feel guilty about wanting to feel normal. Somehow, many of us believe that life should be a struggle, and that if we as patients rise back to health, it has to be under our own power, tugging on our own bootstraps. I'm not sure where we get this philosophy, but I'm sure that it isn't entirely sensible. Why feel guilty for feeling good? If you are one of those people who feels guilty about feeling healthy and energized, discuss this with your counselor, minister, bartender, or whomever you trust. Come back to this book when you are ready to stop feeling bad. Now, let's begin looking at treatments for your fatigue with the one that is the most difficult to convince patients to use.

Traditional Treatments: Medications

"But I don't want to take drugs. Don't you have an herb or vitamin instead?" This sentence has echoed through my head for twelve years, and I always meet it with a big sigh and a smile. I then cue up my mental tape player for a speech that goes something like this:

The medications that we use to treat chemical deficiencies do their job in a very simple way. They are not fake or synthetic neurotransmitters, but rather very simple coenzymes (substances that speed or slow enzymes) that put the brakes on monoamine oxidase, the enzyme that breaks down the neurotransmitters too quickly. This allows the particular neurohormones—either serotonin, norepinephrine, or dopamine—to build back up and return to original levels. No "high," no "happy pill," and no hidden effects or addictions are possible.

Because these medications are chemical compounds, they certainly can cause side effects—but so can any herb or vitamin. Additionally, milk frequently triggers diarrhea, strawberries occasionally cause a rash, and peanuts, in rare circumstances, can cause death. Anything foreign to your body, from breast milk to Budweiser, can affect you in a negative way. Amazingly, compared to must drugs, the compounds that we use to treat fatigue actually cause few side effects.

Without any way to test for it, getting a correct picture of which neurotransmitter is low can be difficult. I always warn patients that my educated guesses on the subject are only that: guesses. But I also tell them that if a significant side effect occurs from the first medication I give them, there is no need to worry—it's not going to harm them and it shouldn't last long. Knowing the symptoms of each neurochemical deficit and understanding the available medications gives experienced practitioners at least a 75 percent chance of finding the right medicine the first time—an average that is increasing all the time, as new research becomes available.

Four current antidepressant medications have the best potential to treat fatigue. In some cases, combinations of these four can be used rather than just one alone. Prozac, the oldest of the group of medicines called SSRI's, works its magic primarily in the serotonin system, the area of the brain where Fibromyalgia and other types of neurotransmitter-induced fatigue can originate. As I mentioned in Chapter Six, there are at least twenty subtypes of serotonin, some of which definitely affect your energy and motivation. Prozac can raise these levels of those types of serotonin and bring about a feeling of wholeness in many people, pulling them out of their beds and back into life. No one knows exactly which serotonin molecules Prozac stimulates, but rival drugs such as Zoloft, Paxil, Lexapro, and Celexa are not known for their energy-lifting abilities. Though the latter do a great job calming the anxious patient, they don't seem to stimulate any get-up-and-go in my patients.

Prozac and its generic version, known as fluoxetine, can be easily combined with other medications and does not have the lurid side effects many seem to think it does. Stories of Prozac patients becoming homicidal or suicidal are ludicrous and unfounded. All that came about because a poorly researched editorial got some sensational press seven or eight years ago; at the time, the FDA investigated and sent letters to all doctors regarding the continued safety of the drug. The damage, however, had been done, and many people today still think that Prozac is a drug for crazy people. Nothing could be further from the truth. I find it to be a cornerstone of treatment in helping fatigued people get their energy back and depressed people get their lives back. Often, they need only take the medicine temporarily, for six months to two years, depending on the seriousness of their symptoms. And as a bonus, it is neither addictive nor habit forming.

Effexor is another medicine that I use to treat fatigue. It's a re-uptake inhibitor of both serotonin and norepinephrine; you can check back in The

Neurotransmitters section of Chapter Six to refresh yourself on the re-uptake process. Effexor increases both norepinephrine and serotonin in the brain and blocks their demise by putting the brakes on the enzymes that break them down. This medicine is often a first choice in treating Fibromyalgia and fatigue. It has been theorized that Effexor works so well because it hits two different neurotransmitters, but some believe that it is just a darn good serotonin medication and that simply causes energy levels to explode. Like Prozac, it is very agreeable to many people who try it, especially when started at 37.5 milligrams for one week, increased to 75 milligrams for another week, and then leveled off at 150 milligrams. Effexor is also known to have less sexual side effects (loss of libido, that sort of thing) than Prozac and its other competitors. I probably prescribe more Effexor for tired patients than all the other medications combined.

A new drug called Cymbalta, acts similarly to Effexor in that it also stimulates the rise of serotonin and norepinephrine. It has just recently become available in the U.S., and I have prescribed it for about fifty of my patients so far. I also offer it as a backup plan if other medicines fail. In further works, I hope to write more about this medicine, but for now, all I can really tell you is that it is very new, and it is safe to take.

The fourth neurotransmitter-altering medicine we'll look at here is Wellbutrin, a potent stimulator of dopamine. I estimate that 30 to 40 percent of people with fatigue need dopamine, either by itself or in combination with another neurotransmitter. Just as exercise can raise serotonin levels, activities such as gambling, drug and nicotine use, viewing pornography, and marathon-level, long distance running all raise dopamine levels by blocking the monoamine oxidase. All things considered, taking a pill is probably a better way to take care of that problem.

Wellbutrin is also sold under the trade name Zyban, which is often used by smokers to break their habit. In patients who are addicted to nicotine or any of the other dopamine stimulators mentioned above, Wellbutrin can raise the levels of dopamine so that the addictive substances or behaviors are not needed. This has certainly been proven effective for nicotine dependency and is currently being tested with drug addicts. Because

Wellbutrin is a potent energy stimulator, possible side effects include sweating, increased pulse, and anxiety—similar to those of too much caffeine. Thankfully, only a small number of patients experience these side effects, which wear off quickly. Some experts used to think that Wellbutrin caused seizures, and it still carries that warning on its package insert. Don't be alarmed, though, because long-term use has proven that seizure rates in people taking Wellbutrin are about the same as they are in people who are not taking medications.

So, which of these pills are right for you? If you smoke, or if you have many blood relatives who smoke (especially Mom and Dad), try Wellbutrin first. Although Effexor can stimulate a little dopamine at high doses, all tobacco-hungry persons owe it to themselves to try Wellbutrin first.

Those of you who aren't fond of cigarettes should probably try Effexor first, due to the dual neurotransmitter stimulation it provides. As previously noted, it stops the breakdown of both serotonin and norepinephrine, making it an excellent drug for mild to moderate anxiety, as well as for depression and fatigue. However, those of you who suffer from panic attacks should have your doctor control your panic symptoms with another agent first! (For my patients with that problem, I prescribe Lexapro, Paxil, or Zoloft before utilizing Effexor, Wellbutrin, or Prozac). Psychiatrists and doctors sometimes mistakenly try to raise energy before controlling the panic and anxiety, but that's like hitting your car's gas pedal before grabbing the steering wheel. It's just not very safe.

Those who don't respond to either Effexor or Cymbalta should give Prozac a try—especially if they have a lot of anxiety issues as well. Maximum dosage can usually be pushed as high as 80 milligrams, though usually 40 suffices. Prozac also comes in a once-weekly formulation, for those who dislike taking medication every day. The chief side effect of Prozac is sexual in nature, with both men and women having increased difficulty in achieving orgasm. About 30 percent of people taking Prozac experience this to varying degrees. If the drug is working well for you and you do have a problem with these sexual side effects, try some over-the-counter Ginseng supplements. Interestingly, because Wellbutrin is the only of the drugs we're looking at that has no sexual side effects, it is occasionally added to get rid of them when they are caused by the other medications.

Combination Therapy

As hinted at in the last section, it is sometimes necessary to blend a couple of medicines to achieve a complete relief of fatigue, similar to the way antibiotics are frequently paired to treat a complex infection. Except for mixing Effexor and Cymbalta (they are in the same family of dual-mechanism drugs), the above medicines can all be mixed with one another because they each hit different neurotransmitters. If you are already on an antidepressant other than those above, the general rule is that you can add any of the above to the current drug, as long as it is in another family—that is, as long as it doesn't affect the same neurotransmitter that's already being affected by the medication you are currently taking. For example, Wellbutrin, Cymbalta, or Effexor could be added to any other antidepressant (the rest of which are all serotonin medicines, such as Celexa, Lexapro, Zoloft or Paxil) because they hail from different families. Doctors tend not to blend two drugs from the same family, such as Zoloft and Prozac, unless it's a fairly desperate situation.

One unique blend, which is the brainchild of Dr. Steven Stahl (the "Father of Neurotransmitters") is Effexor and a drug called Remeron. This latter antidepressant increases levels of the neurochemical norepinephrine in the blood and thus boosts energy. This combo has been nicknamed the "California Rocket" by those who use it.

Blending medications is not only essential for treating simultaneous anxiety and fatigue, as previously mentioned, but it is also sometimes necessary to bolster your energy. Usually, if you have no side effects from one medicine, adding a second drug rarely creates new side effects. Because 20 to 30 percent of people with fatigue have two or more neurotransmitter deficiencies, combining agents may be the only way to help them completely.

Other Medications

Sometimes, people using the above methods don't improve completely, or in some cases, not at all. If this is your case, and your doctor is sure that there are no other medical causes of your fatigue, there are some other "tricks" he can use. Psychiatrists frequently try Ritalin, a stimulant usually reserved for ADHD to boost dopamine levels. Family doctors are a bit shy about using this drug outside of ADHD, due to its abuse potential; usually, a psychiatric referral is needed to prescribe it, often with good reason. The complexity of the neurotransmitter system can confuse many health professionals and it's not a bad idea to get a psychiatric consult to assure that all medicines blend appropriately and hold a reasonable chance of working.

Provigil is another medicine that can add energy, especially if narcolepsy is suspected. (It was designed for B-1 bomber pilots to stay energized on long missions, without making them jittery ... interesting, no?) I have prescribed it, however, for many of my fatigued patients who do not have sleeping disorders. The side effects are usually minimal and the drug is safe, though expensive—at $200 a month, I can see why insurance companies complain about it. But if this is the only medicine that can give you back your life, who could argue with that?

Natural Hormones

The word "natural" makes my stomach twist into knots. Not that there is anything wrong with nature, mind you; it's just that the word is abused more than the American taxpayer. Natural means "found in nature," and anything in nature must be good for you, right? Like arsenic, or cyanide—get the picture?

Natural hormones are hormone-like substances that are found in plants and can act in the body the way testosterone, estrogen, and progesterone do. As our own hormone levels sink with age, occasionally fatigue can be a result. Manufactured testosterone, available as a patch, cream, or injection can bring back the vigor in men with low levels. The woman's choices, however, are not as desirable. Women's synthetic hormones are at the root of weight gain, depression, blood clots, strokes, heart attacks, and breast cancer.

So, natural hormones, especially for women, have become pretty popular. Although I have no results of specific studies to share with you, I do know some women who have tried these harmless substances and have seemed to get more energy, calmness, and symptom control during menopause. Some researchers even believe that the progesterone creams can help lower rates of breast cancer, and from what I have seen myself, I have to say that I agree.

Finding someone to test the levels of "natural" hormones in your body can be difficult, because there is still a lot of controversy surrounding these compounds. Powerful drug companies are not interested in losing sales to these new competitors, so prepare for some scoffing. Women wanting more information can look up zrtlabs.com on the World Wide Web for a list of local experts who may be able to help. For men, your doctor should perform blood levels of total and free testosterone if you have lost your sex drive or upper musculature. Prescription therapy is available to treat this condition.

Herbal Supplements

Though I mentioned them before, let me reiterate some thoughts regarding this multibillion-dollar industry. I had an opportunity not long ago to attend a conference on herbs, vitamins, and supplements, co-sponsored by Harvard Medical School and UCSF. Designed for primary care providers, the conference was a forum of doctors, pharmacists, and an herbalist or two who together discussed alternative therapies for patients. Expecting to go home with a notebook full of new treatments to pass on to my patients, I was terribly disappointed to find out that American herbs, though possibly tasting good sprinkled over a Cornish hen, fall flat as medical therapy. They are just too weak.

England, on the other hand, sells herbs at full potency, and physicians who know exactly how and why they work control their distribution. When our U.S. Congress enacted legislation to allow over the counter sales of these substances, they gave the FDA a policing role in choosing the potency. Under a great deal of pressure from lobbyists, the FDA decided to sell watered down doses over the counter, rather than restrict access with prescriptions. Because these herbs cannot exceed near-homeopathic levels, most of them are, in a word, weak.

In an attempt to remedy the potency problem, companies try mixing multiple herbs that have similar effects, but ten impotent doses of ten mixed drugs still gets you nowhere. The good news is that, for the most part, if taken as directed, the herbs seem to be fairly safe. But remember that they are still drugs, no different from ones sold by prescription, so talk to your pharmacist or doctor if you are going to add an herb to your daily regimen, especially if you are on prescription medication.

Honestly, if your goal is to add energy to your life, herbs are not a choice I recommend. My one exception is DHEA, which we discussed in Chapter Five; it may help with sex drive and energy some people. Any doctor can check levels of DHEA easily in the bloodstream.

Vitamins

So, if herbs aren't much help with fatigue, are vitamins any better? Well ... no. Although vitamins are necessary substances found in foods and sunlight, the rumor of their widespread depletion in humans is greatly exaggerated. For some medical conditions, vitamins are prescribed appropriately—hair loss, osteoporosis, leg cramps, and so on. And I usually recommend a cheap multivitamin for those who don't eat properly or who have intestinal diseases that prevent them from absorbing the vitamins correctly. Beyond that, not one clinical study shows any benefit from using vitamins to treat fatigue. Yet billions of dollars' worth of these agents are purchased and consumed each year.

After thinking long and hard for several years on the subject, I've decided that three things play a role in making vitamins so inviting:

1. They're easy to get and take. Other than some of the horse-sized ones, vitamins are easily dispensed, don't need a prescription, and are fairly affordable.

2. They're an excellent way to rebel against the forces of traditional medicine. This is especially true if the problem that you face isn't life threatening. Because of modern medicine's less than perfect past, patients love to find alternative therapies to cure their ailments. Being able to choose your own therapy without the controlling oversight of a doctor can feed your rebellious nature. And I can deal with that, being a bit of a rebel myself. Just don't be a rebel without a cause.

3. Vitamins are mysterious. People love mystery—what's behind door number three, blind dates, lottery tickets—it's a common human trait to wonder what might happen. "Perhaps these pills will give me energy and make me stronger," people think. And with vitamin names like "Mega-man," can't you see the attraction? If you can see the attraction, just keep in mind that all vitamins except A, D, E, and K are water soluble, meaning that most of whatever you're taking will wash right out of your body. Any amount greater than what your body needs will go straight into your urine; the magic and mystery will melt away as your hundred dollar-per-month vitamins stream into the toilet.

So, you see, vitamins and herbs do not really have much of a role in treating fatigue, other than the small job of maintaining overall health—and that's accomplished merely with the amount of vitamins we get in our food. If my criticism seems harsh, I apologize. I get frustrated watching so many patients waste not only their money, but precious moments of their lives; they are taking vitamins and living with fatigue when better therapies exist. The way I see it, if you want to reject scientific discovery as a basis for making your life better, then be consistent—stay off airplanes and out of automobiles, stop watching TV, and don't even think of using my pager number next time you need an antibiotic! Not going to happen, is it? Okay, so let's look at some real non-drug methods of getting back your energy.

Alternative Ideas:
Diet And Metabolism

Oh, sweet Buddha ... not the "D" word! Yes friends, I'm afraid so—it's time to talk about your diet. Beyond a healthy diet for a healthy body, diet relates to fatigue in another way. Namely, it's Metabolic Syndrome, something I mentioned way back in Chapter Four. It's a fairly unknown condition of insulin resistance that is a precursor to Diabetes, and it frequently causes fatigue and weakness, but it can be remedied with proper diet. To understand the hows and whys, let's first take a quick look at how certain foods can cause our weariness.

When carbohydrates—starches such as potatoes, bread, and sugar—are consumed, they break down into simple sugars that are only needed by your body in small amounts. When this sugar hits the bloodstream via the stomach and small intestine, the level of sweetness in your blood begins to rise. The pancreas, your body's thermostat for sugar levels, releases insulin in response to the higher level of sugar. Insulin picks up the sugar and takes it to muscle cells all over the body—we covered this back in Chapter Four as well. Once it arrives, the insulin helps the glucose (sugar) into the cell, where it can be used for energy. I sometimes use the example of the insulin cop arresting the sugar criminal and taking him to the muscle cell jail. When this works well, insulin levels remain low and the body is happy.

Trouble comes to town with the onset of Metabolic Syndrome, a gradual condition of insulin resistance by the muscle cell. The cause of this "rusting" of the jail door can be genetics (do you have any Diabetic family members?), obesity, lack of exercise, or a combination of any of the three. The muscle cells begin to open their doors less freely, causing the sugar levels to rise in the bloodstream. The pancreas senses this elevation and releases a double dose of insulin, hoping to find enough "well-oiled doors" through which to slide the sugar. As long as enough doors are found, your body can get the sugar levels down to a normal range, which is between 60 and 125. So, everything is fine then ... right?

Not really. As the insulin levels continue to rise over the years, they have a profound effect on the body. A tiny amount of insulin was sufficient when we were young, but larger quantities are necessary as we get older and less fit. The pancreas begins to work overtime and weekends to crank out enough insulin to store away the sugar, while we obliviously gulp down another soda and super-sized order of fries.

The problems come when we start feeling how high levels of insulin can ravage our bodies. Besides debilitating fatigue, the elevated pancreatic hormone causes increased fat absorption, weight gain, and a slower metabolism. We were never meant to have this level of insulin in the body, and it drags us down; as we continue to put on weight and slow down, we become more insulin resistant. And that's how we wake up one day 15 or 150 pounds overweight and too tired to do anything about it.

Are you insulin resistant? Could a change in diet increase your energy levels? Let's look at some clues about Metabolic Syndrome and fatigue and try to find some answers to those questions.

First, insulin resistance typically (not always, just typically) follows a genetic line. Diabetes in close relatives strongly raises your chances of getting Metabolic Syndrome. Second, do you exercise on a regular basis? As I mentioned a few paragraphs ago, physical activity "oils the hinges" on the muscle cells' doors and makes it easier to get the sugar inside, which keeps your insulin levels low. Third, do you have a weight problem? I'm not talking about you 105-pounders who freak out after gaining a pound. I'm talking about a spare tire, or perhaps a few spare tires that are dragging you down. Lastly, do you get sleepy after a high-carbohydrate meal? If the answer is yes to any of these questions, you may have Metabolic Syndrome and could benefit from a healthy, low-carbohydrate diet.

Blood work is the easiest way to tell if you suffer from insulin resistance or Metabolic Syndrome. Cholesterol levels usually rise because of the higher levels of insulin coursing through your body, though your HDL ("good cholesterol") levels usually will be lower than normal. Fasting insulin levels, which are drawn in the morning, before you eat breakfast, usually show elevated insulin due to the pancreas' working around the clock to lower the sugar. Lastly, an HgA1C test—a four-month average of blood sugars—will help determine how insulin resistant you are. In that test, a larger number means a higher average sugar, and the higher the insulin level will be. Numbers less than 5.5 are fairly normal, 5.6 to 6.1 are insulin resistant, and greater than 6.1 has crossed over into Diabetes.

For those of you who may be resistant—and if you are, welcome to 30 percent of the American population—diet and exercise can really help. Because carbohydrates (especially the simple starches that break down quickly) turn into sugar, avoiding them will force insulin levels to drop. When this happens, metabolism and energy rebound. Exercise, of course, also helps lower the resistance and lessens the need for insulin. This also releases energy and causes weight loss.

The wars over low carbohydrate diets have been waged and debated endlessly. Do I pass on the pasta? Do I frown at the fruit? Are there good carbohydrates? Tough questions, but I'll try to give you some simple answers.

Yes, there are good and bad carbohydrates. And by enjoying the good ones and shunning the bad, you can revive your energy, get control of your weight problem, and improve your health. The way to tell a good carbohydrate from a bad one is to check its glycemic index. Low glycemic index carbohydrates break down slowly and don't blast up insulin levels, because the sugar they release at any one moment is small. High glycemic carbohydrates turn rapidly to sugar, causing insulin to be dumped into the bloodstream—you guessed it—rapidly. The South Beach Diet, the best book I could recommend to learn more about the glycemic index, lists the foods that are in each category. For those of you who have Type II Diabetes, insulin resistance, or just trouble controlling your weight, I think it is probably the best resource available at the time of this writing.

Typically, your energy level rises when on a lower carbohydrate diet, and excess weight usually drops. For those of you who cannot exercise for whatever reason, your doctor may prescribe Metformin, a drug that oils those rusty hinges on the muscle cell doors for you. This can help jump-start the process of lowering your insulin levels the way exercise might. Though typically a Diabetic medicine, doctors actually use it in Metabolic Syndrome to ward off Diabetes and induce weight loss.

By eating healthy foods, avoiding high fat, and avoiding high glycemic carbohydrates, you can maximize your body function, stave off Diabetes, and enjoy good health. Because fatigue is multi-factorial, diet plays an important role in combating it.

Exercise

Although I briefly mentioned it above, this topic is so important to treating fatigue that I have to give it its own section as well. I already know what you're thinking, though: "If I could exercise, I wouldn't be fatigued!" I understand, and you are right. But hear me out, and I am sure we can come to a compromise.

Besides improving insulin resistance and lowering the fatigue producing hormone (that would be insulin), exercise helps build neurotransmitters in the brain. Serotonin, norepinephrine, and dopamine all increase after the implementation of a steady, regular exercise program. As mentioned prior, neurotransmitter deficiency is by far the number one cause of fatigue that I see. And aerobic exercise is a great way to combat it.

I realize that because of various disabilities, some of you may not be able to implement this "tool" as fully as you would like to. But usually some form of exercise—think about swimming, water therapy, walking, arm exercises, or riding a stationary bike—can be accomplished some degree. Excuses are always easier than solutions so don't let anything hold you back.

Think of an exercise that you can do, in whatever amount you can do it, and just go and do it!

As for frequency of exercising, try working your way up to at least thirty minutes of aerobic conditioning, five or six days per week. I know that not everyone will be able to do that, but keep in mind that even weightlifting (be it light hand weights or heavy barbells) can become aerobic if you don't rest more than thirty seconds between sets and you keep your heart rate at an appropriate level. Of course, first ask your doctor if an exercise regimen is safe for you and what heart rate range you should be in during exercise. And once you have begun, don't fall into the trap of doing the same routine. The body learns to adapt quickly, so change your workout occasionally to keep yourself interested and wanting to do more.

Lastly, I want to say something to those of you who use lack of time as an excuse to not exercise. Stop lying to yourself! You may not take the time, but you have it. Perhaps becoming more creative about a solution would help, like using equipment at home while you watch your kids or your favorite TV program. Or maybe you need to make exercise more fun, so that you will want to find time to do it; you know that something you find boring will not last for long. Personally, I listen to upbeat music and watch sports highlights on cable while I exercise—it takes my mind off the fact that really, I hate to exercise. Maybe you need to find a new racquetball partner, mix things up on the court and make it a little more challenging. You need to think and be creative to find the right exercise program for you. You may not conquer your fatigue completely if you don't.

Yoga

No, I don't fold up like a pretzel either. But millions of people are learning to unleash the power within by utilizing this time-tested practice. Yoga is a complex set of breathing exercises and movements designed to put the body and mind into harmony. Though originally rooted in the Hindu tradition, most yoga participants in the West don't subscribe to the particular religious teachings. Like meditation, it can augment religion or be completely separate. It is not mystical or magical, but it follows good medical principles regarding the inner workings of the body.

In Chapter Five, I described how stress increases monoamine oxidase activity in the brain, lowering our neurotransmitters. Yoga seems to decrease cortisol production and lower monoamine oxidase activity; the result is an increase in neurotransmitters and the energy that comes with it. It may be used as an adjunct to medicines or exercise, or perhaps, practiced by itself. Although some patients report as much success with yoga as with medicines, I recommend that you do not stop your prescriptions without talking to your doctor. And if you are just starting yoga, realize that you will need to practice it for a while (at least six to eight weeks) before seeing the neurotransmitter benefits.

When done regularly, yoga can be a great way to raise your neurotransmitter level and fight your fatigue. Classes abound at local YMCA's, gyms, churches, and schools. Videos are also available for those who wish to practice in the privacy of their home. The small amount of invested time will pay off in mental clarity, energy, relaxation, and health. I recommend that you try it and be patient, as new things take time to sink into your brain and insinuate change.

Meditation

Like Yoga, anything that battles stress helps us battle fatigue—and most of us just don't know how stressed we truly are. Meditation can help ease stress, both perceived (the stuff we know about) and subconscious (the stuff we don't recognize or admit to). A variety of methods are available but beyond the scope of this book. There are multiple written volumes on the subject of meditation, and a trip to your local bookstore should prove useful if you want to learn more about it.

For those of you with religious roots, I'll mention that the meditation I am writing about is not based on spiritual teachings, but rather sound, psychological principles. For many, regular prayer (to any deity) can bring similar benefits. Both disciplines quiet the mind by focusing it on something outside of itself. Freeing ourselves from negative thinking, eloping from our helter-skelter lifestyles and shielding the brain from constant stimulation helps us promote neurotransmitter rebound. By focusing on our breathing and other bodily centers, we learn to let go, reducing the action of monoamine oxidase, and therefore our fatigue. Psychologists are usually a good source of information on meditation and can show you how to proceed.

Cognitive Therapy

It may seem a little out of the ordinary, but I'm serious—cognitive therapy is a method of combating fatigue, though it should be used along with one of the other treatments we've been looking at here. It seems to work best for Chronic Fatigue Syndrome, where constant weariness over long periods of time leads to reactive patterns of thought that are reactive—meaning, you're so tired that all you can think about is being tired. This in turn lowers neurotransmitters and produces more tiredness. Defining your fears, exploring your subconscious mind, and illuminating your "dark side" can block monoamine oxidase and help you build precious neurohormones. Though it can be time consuming, and expensive, it has a sound medical and psychological basis and can play a role in finding your energy. Anyone with a traumatic past, especially victims of rape, abuse, or other violence, owes it to themselves to consider trying cognitive therapy with a trained psychologist. Your primary doctor can refer you to someone with the proper credentials.

Hypnotism

Though a little unconventional, and definitely not the first therapy I think about when discussing fatigue, hypnotism can help restore neurotransmitter function in the brain the way that yoga, meditation, and cognitive therapy do. Not all patients respond to this interesting treatment, but I do know that some of my patients have found it successful. So if other therapies don't work for you, why not try it?

Hobbies

All of us need to do things that we enjoy to pass the time. No, beer drinking and "the art of the remote" are not hobbies—they may be more of a way of life. A hobby is something that interests you, something in which you can invest yourself. So, how does this possibly combat fatigue? And where are you going to find the energy to engage in a hobby?

Like many of the other suggestions for getting back your energy, some effort is required for this one. But the rewards can be tremendous! Once again, I am looking for ways to elevate neurotransmitters. Here is my take on the subject.

Somehow, our society has equated our work with our worth. We drown ourselves in jobs, businesses, bills, bank accounts, and a host of other things. We unbalance ourselves, which leads to neurotransmitter deficiency. Engaging in enjoyable hobbies relaxes us, thus reducing the actions of monoamine oxidase. They don't need to be high-energy activities like mountain biking or rock climbing, but it does need to be something that you truly enjoy and that doesn't stress you out.

Before you leap into an activity, take some time to think about what you want to do. If a hobby becomes boring, it becomes work. If it becomes work, it will pull down your neurotransmitters. In all probability, an idea is not going to jump out at you at this moment. And the whole thing may sound ludicrous to you right now. But be patient, and I promise you, it will come around.

I believe that every one of us has a talent, or a gift—whatever you call that seemingly innate ability to do certain things. Because we generally enjoy what we do well, these gifts point us toward possible hobbies, if we let them. But many things may hold us back. Maybe some of us feel that we owe our time to others—children, spouses, or bosses, to name a few. Maybe we feel that painting or writing is wasting time, not contributing anything useful to the world. Maybe we feel the need to show productivity to the "time police" at the end of the day, thereby justifying our existence. Boy, are we screwed up! Hobbies aren't a waste of time. They are an investment of time. By concentrating on doing things we enjoy, our minds become fresher and more productive for when we do go back to work or back to our families.

For those of you still struggling over which hobby to pursue, ask your friends and family to tell you about your strengths and talents. Also, think back to when you were a kid. What did you love to do? What did you do well? What did your friends say you did well?

Hobbies can help balance out and bring meaning to our lives. Hobbies don't need to produce anything or be functional in any way. For all I care, you can paint a scene, and then paint right back over it. It's just that we need harmony between our working and our living. Denying our need to achieve balance will deny us the energy we need to run our lives.

The Combination Method

Fighting fatigue, as you can see, is a multidisciplinary task, usually requiring more than one therapy. Hollywood, magazines, and over-hyped infomercials make us believe that somewhere out there, a panacea exists. People cram into my office week after week, convinced that they have an abnormality that I can cure with a wave of my magic wand. Sadly, we all know that that just isn't going to happen.

The road back to energetic health comes with commitment, fight, and a blueprint for your return. If you can raise your own neuro-hormonal levels, you can find your fountain of youthful energy. But it doesn't always come easily. Three things you should most definitely do:

1. Assure no other medical illness exists

2. Look at possible medication use to jumpstart your neurotransmitters

3. Use time-tested, non-pharmacological techniques, like exercise and meditation

You should also fight every demon that begs you to lie down. Try out at least one of the activities we just talked about—yoga, therapy, a hobby. We go about our hectic lives, forgetting each day that we are dynamic beings, not static ones. We plod along and we forget the one common denominator that prevails through the whole process of living: our senses of self. By identifying the unreasonable demands that we place on ourselves, finding ways to commune with our inner beings, and treating the genetically acquired and stress-induced depletion of neurotransmitters, we can find our way through the dark forest of fatigue and walk into the meadow of a brand new day.

Put It All Together

So, did you make it through the forest? Or did you trip on the complicated medical vines that seemed to run in every direction? In this chapter, I will explain the tests that you should have your doctor order, summarize the diseases that cause fatigue, and help you devise an exit strategy for your fatigue. So grab a pen, sharpen up your sword of reason, and let's slay this dragon once and for all.

Blood Work

Every fatigued person should get some basic blood testing done to screen out diseases that are more serious. Here are the bare essentials that primary care providers must perform:

- CBC (Complete Blood Count)
- Chem Profile (liver, kidney, electrolytes, sugar, proteins and more)
- TSH, Free T3, and T4 (full thyroid profile)
- ESR (erythrocyte sedimentation rate—a measure of inflammation in the blood and body)

This basic series of tests covers most diseases. But if you're a discriminating medical shopper, what else should your testing include? Let's skim our way back across the tops of the trees and find out what other investigations should be considered. Keep a list of those things that strike a chord with your symptoms or physical signs, so that you can talk about them with your medical provider.

Other Lab Testing:
Endocrine

It's hard to ignore the effects of hormones on the body, and I think for the first time, saliva testing (for women, mostly) may answer some questions that previously kept doctors scratching their heads. Special tests on the saliva, looking for estrogen toxicity, progesterone deficiency, and DHEA levels, seem reasonable—although the science is still in its infancy. These tests should only be performed after a thorough investigation by a primary care provider has been performed. You can find more information about saliva testing at zrtlabs.com.

Other hormone blood tests that your doctor might perform are FSH and LH (pituitary hormones) for women who may be in or near menopause. Men should have testosterone (both total and free levels) checked, especially if their fatigue is accompanied by a lack of sex drive or upper body strength loss. Men with strong libidos need not get this test.

If your weight has increased with your fatigue, you should consider having fasting insulin and fasting cortisol tests done. These tests check for Metabolic Syndrome and Cushing's disease, respectively. For those who are concerned about Diabetes, an HgA1C test will show an average blood sugar for the last four months. For the folks thinking that their sugar is low, remember that hypoglycemia only causes temporary fatigue, not constant weariness.

Infection

If you have a low-grade fever that doesn't have any readily visible cause and lasts longer than three weeks, you may have an infection somewhere in your body. If you think this is your problem, have blood cultures done. In this test, blood is taken from your arm, put it in a special lab dish, and used to grow bacteria. The kind of bacteria that grows indicates the location of the infection in your body. For example, if your blood culture shows certain bacteria that are known to grow in the heart, you'd know that that is where your infection is hiding.

HIV and hepatitis B and C are viral infections that can be real energy pillagers. Tests for them should be run on anyone with a history of unprotected sex, indiscriminate needle usage, blood transfusions before 1986, alcohol or drug abuse, or anyone working with bodily fluids, such as people in the medical profession.

Though fungi (such as molds and yeast) can grow in the body, these types of infections are not very common. Blood work is a poor way to find them, but chest x-rays usually are good. Chronic fungus infections can also be seen at times in the skin and sinus tract.

Cardiac

Heart ailments are frequently detected by your doctor's basic stethoscope and by an EKG. However, for a stronger diagnosis, tests such as a stress thallium scan or ultrasound can be done. Any patient with chest pain, a family history of heart ailments, or shortness of breath or fatigue after exertion, needs cardiac testing. Patients who wake up feeling good but tire out faster than they used to also need to have a serious work up on their cardiac system. For those who cannot walk enough for a stress test, ask for a Persantine stress test. That one can be done lying down.

Pulmonary

Everyone over the age of 35 who is fatigued with no readily discernible cause should have a chest x-ray performed. If you also have shortness of breath, a pulmonary function study would be reasonable. In this test, a technician measures your ability to suck and blow on a tube; it may sound silly, but it may help unmask restrictive and obstructive diseases of the lungs. However, unless you have persistent shortness of breath along with your fatigue, these tests probably are not necessary.

If you wake up tired, go to bed tired, and fall asleep easily in between, consider sleep testing. Patients who are sleepy and tired all day, but don't fall asleep, probably don't have sleep apnea, but for those who do, something called a CPAP machine can give your life back. Sleep apnea is fairly common; I diagnose two or three cases of it per month. People with daytime drowsiness but normal sleep study results should consider a blood test for narcolepsy (HLA antigens) to help rule out or rule in the disease. But of course, if you have any questions about your condition, see a sleep doctor before you go through with any of these tests.

Orthopedic

Orthopedists don't help us a whole lot when it comes to fatigue, but let's not disregard them. Anyone after the age of fifty with fatigue and bone pain should get x-rays of their painful areas or a bone scan, to rule out Paget's disease.

Neurological

Anyone fatigued person who feels more weak than tired—for example, you can't grip your coffee cup well, or get out of a chair easily—may need a good neurological exam, complete with strength and reflex grading. Any regular doctor can perform this exam. However, if your primary doctor suspects nerve or muscular disease, you should get an EMG done. Rarely, an MRI of the brain, a spinal tap, or an EEG (brainwave scan) is necessary for fatigued patients.

Rheumatological

The biggest help a rheumatologist can provide is a diagnosis of Fibromyalgia, which, as you know, has no definitive testing. Blood testing can also rule out other rheumatic diseases. A rheumatoid profile screens for Lupus and Rheumatoid Arthritis; you can also get a test to rule out Lyme disease, a rare but possible cause of fatigue and joint pain. Remember that neurotransmitter deficiency frequently causes body pain with fatigue, so don't over diagnose your discomfort in light of normal blood test results.

Everything Else

All other bodily systems can be checked by the standard blood tests mentioned at the beginning of this chapter, such as hematologic (anemias), GI (gastrointestinal), and renal (kidney).

What It All Comes Down To

The human body is an amazing collection of complex interactions; it makes the space shuttle look like a paper airplane in comparison. The billions upon billions of chemical reactions that occur each minute inside our bodies allow us to tune into the world around us—imbibing its fragrance, feeling its color, and hearing its song.

The scourge of fatigue takes us away from that world and into dark bedrooms. We curl up with blankets rather than nature, and we curse the birds for waking us up with their songs. The price of weariness is astronomical, even before you calculate its toll on our spirits. It is my belief that most fatigue is conquerable, and it was my intention to blaze a trail through the thick forests of human physiology, anatomy, and pathology, in hopes that you might follow and gain some insight. I trust that I didn't leave you in a thicket.

You have a right as a rider on this planet to live your life with vigor. I encourage you to take your discoveries, notes, and questions and seek help from a qualified primary physician. If your requests for testing are blown off, trade your doctor in for one who listens to you when you talk. If you are uninsured, find a clinic in your area that can get the tests covered by a grant or other social program. Local teaching hospitals are good sources. Don't waste another day trapped by exhaustion. You deserve better.

Notes